MW00565116

Yoga and Meditation at the Library

PRACTICAL GUIDES FOR LIBRARIANS

⊚ About the Series

This innovative series written and edited for librarians by librarians provides authoritative, practical information and guidance on a wide spectrum of library processes and operations.

Books in the series are focused, describing practical and innovative solutions to a problem facing today's librarian and delivering step-by-step guidance for planning, creating, implementing, managing, and evaluating a wide range of services and programs.

The books are aimed at beginning and intermediate librarians needing basic instruction/guidance in a specific subject and at experienced librarians who need to gain knowledge in a new area or guidance in implementing a new program/service.

⊚ About the Series Editors

The **Practical Guides for Librarians** series was conceived and edited by M. Sandra Wood, MLS, MBA, AHIP, FMLA, Librarian Emerita, Penn State University Libraries from 2014-2017.

M. Sandra Wood was a librarian at the George T. Harrell Library, the Milton S. Hershey Medical Center, College of Medicine, Pennsylvania State University, Hershey, PA, for over thirty-five years, specializing in reference, educational, and database services. Ms. Wood received an MLS from Indiana University and an MBA from the University of Maryland. She is a fellow of the Medical Library Association and served as a member of MLA's Board of Directors from 1991 to 1995.

Ellyssa Kroski assumed editorial responsibilities for the series beginning in 2017. She is the director of Information Technology at the New York Law Institute as well as an award-winning editor and author of 36 books including *Law Librarianship in the Digital Age* for which she won the AALL's 2014 Joseph L. Andrews Legal Literature Award. Her ten-book technology series, *The Tech Set* won the ALA's Best Book in Library Literature Award in 2011. Ms. Kroski is a librarian, an adjunct faculty member at Drexel and San Jose State University, and an international conference speaker. She has just been named the winner of the 2017 Library Hi Tech Award from the ALA/LITA for her long-term contributions in the area of Library and Information Science technology and its application.

1. *How to Teach: A Practical Guide for Librarians* by Beverley E. Crane
2. *Implementing an Inclusive Staffing Model for Today's Reference Services* by Julia K. Nims, Paula Storm, and Robert Stevens
3. *Managing Digital Audiovisual Resources: A Practical Guide for Librarians* by Matthew C. Mariner
4. *Outsourcing Technology: A Practical Guide for Librarians* by Robin Hastings
5. *Making the Library Accessible for All: A Practical Guide for Librarians* by Jane Vincent
6. *Discovering and Using Historical Geographic Resources on the Web: A Practical Guide for Librarians* by Eva H. Dodsworth and L. W. Laliberté

Yoga and Meditation at the Library

A Practical Guide for Librarians

Jenn Carson

PRACTICAL GUIDES FOR LIBRARIANS, NO. 64

ROWMAN & LITTLEFIELD
Lanham • Boulder • New York • London

Published by Rowman & Littlefield

An imprint of The Rowman & Littlefield Publishing Group, Inc.

4501 Forbes Boulevard, Suite 200, Lanham, Maryland 20706

www.rowman.com

6 Tinworth Street, London, SE11 5AL, United Kingdom

Copyright © 2019 by The Rowman & Littlefield Publishing Group, Inc.

All rights reserved. No part of this book may be reproduced in any form or by any electronic or mechanical means, including information storage and retrieval systems, without written permission from the publisher, except by a reviewer who may quote passages in a review.

British Library Cataloguing in Publication Information Available

Library of Congress Cataloging-in-Publication Data

Names: Carson, Jenn, author.

Title: Yoga and meditation at the library : a practical guide for librarians / Jenn Carson.

Description: Lanham : Rowman & Littlefield Publishing Group, 2019. | Series: Practical guides for librarians ; 64 | Includes bibliographical references and index.

Identifiers: LCCN 2018057380 (print) | LCCN 2018060319 (ebook) | ISBN 9781538116883 (Electronic) | ISBN 9781538116876 (pbk. : alk. paper)

Subjects: LCSH: Libraries—Activity programs | Yoga—Study and teaching. | Meditation—Study and teaching.

Classification: LCC Z716.33 (ebook) | LCC Z716.33 .Y64 2019 (print) | DDC 025.5—dc23

LC record available at https://lccn.loc.gov/2018057380

♾™ The paper used in this publication meets the minimum requirements of American National Standard for Information Sciences—Permanence of Paper for Printed Library Materials, ANSI/NISO Z39.48-1992.

Printed in the United States of America

For Janet, who taught me how to sit quietly.

I'm sorry I still have ants in my pants.

Contents

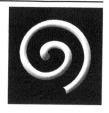

Preface

The Crisis, or Why We Need This Book

Did you know, according to a Gallup poll conducted in 2017, 79 percent of Americans say they feel stress "sometimes" or "frequently" throughout their day?[1] A more comprehensive survey administered by the American Psychological Association in the same year found that Americans' average stress levels were 4.8 (on a scale of 1–10) and found that 75 percent of all survey participants experienced symptoms like anxiety, irritability, or fatigue related to their stress levels in the past month.[2] While these stress levels are pretty high across all generations, millennials (currently age eighteen to thirty-eight) were the most stressed out, with an average stress level of 5.7. And surprisingly, older adults (currently age seventy-two and older) were found to have the sharpest increase in stress, despite being the least stressed population, with an average of 3.3. Health care (or lack thereof) was stated as the number one cause of stress. With our stress levels, growing obesity rates, and the increase in heart disease and chronic illness, clearly our traditional approaches to health care are not working. The World Health Organization (WHO) is warning that our lack of exercise is putting one in four people at risk for serious health conditions like heart disease and diabetes.[3] Our approaches to stress reduction and attempts at preventative health maintenance aren't working either, since the newest generation is more stressed and is predicted to be less healthy than their parents by the time they reach middle age.[4] And this isn't just happening in America. This state of world health (or lack thereof) has hit such a crisis that the WHO added physical activity to its global action mandate in May 2018 in an effort to combat these alarming trends.

A Different Approach to Living, or Librarian-ing

Before you crawl under your desk in despair, wondering what you can possibly do to help with such a widespread and complex issue, know that (thankfully!) libraries have been sitting up and taking notice for a while.[5] For the last decade, I have been offering yoga, meditation, and other movement-based wellness programs in libraries, museums, and classrooms, and I'm not the only one. In 2017, I created a survey that was administered through the American Library Association's member newsletter; of the more than three hundred people who responded, 65 percent said they offered some form of programming that encouraged physical activity.[6] The majority of respondents were from public or school libraries. The most popular offerings were yoga, dance, games, tai chi, martial arts, and gardening activities. Also in 2017, I helped Noah Lenstra from the University of North Carolina, Greensboro, design a survey that was administered to more than fifteen hundred librarians across North America, and the results showed that yoga was by far the most popular program.[7] In 2018, I wrote a book exploring the growing trend of physical literacy in libraries called *Get Your Community Moving: Physical Literacy Programs for All Ages*, which featured interviews with librarians all across North America who are working to make movement-based programs part of daily public library service.[8] Outside the library system, within the general population, there is a growing segment of North Americans who are taking cues from our Eastern neighbors and incorporating more yoga and meditation into their lifestyles, with staggering results. According to a 2012 report on comprehensive health services performed by the National Center for Health Statistics, 8 percent (18 million) of US adults practice meditation and 9.5 percent (21 million) practice yoga, with the numbers growing annually.[9] This is having a trickle-down effect to our children and students, with 1.6 percent (927,000) practicing meditation and 3.1 percent (1.7 million) practicing yoga.[10] It was such impressive results it is *still* making the news, as I just (in November 2018, six years later) saw a report on CNN featuring results from the same investigation.[11] Why is this news? Because yoga and meditation, if you are doing them right, work. And who is better poised to offer free tools that promise to make our lives better in a place that is accessible to everyone, in program formats that can reach across all socioeconomic, cultural, gender, and political divides? No one. The library, especially the public library, is going to be the one to make this happen. We are the living room of the people, and they are going to come sit and stretch with us.

⦿ Inreach, or Bringing It Home

Library staff are not exempt from rising stress levels. According to a 2006 study performed by the British Psychological Society's Division of Occupational Psychology, it was found that among firefighters, police officers, train operators, teachers, and librarians, the librarians ranked the *highest* in the level of perceived occupational stress overall.[12] We're more stressed than people who put out fires for a living! So we also need to get better at tackling our own health and stress-related problems so that we can pass on this information to our patrons, and set healthy examples for our staff and families.

⦿ Exuberance, or the Urge to Play

As librarians and library administrators, we may often tentatively approach program planning hoping to be armed with policies and procedures coming from a quantitative methodology, which is understandable since our funding may largely rely on producing reliable—and hopefully impressive—metrics. Also, as librarians, we have been trained to identify, classify, and catalog information in order to ease access and control chaos. You may have picked up this book because you've been wanting to deliver yoga and meditation programs in your library, but are meeting a lot of resistance from the top, or perhaps even from patrons or colleagues with the belief that movement-based programs shouldn't be part of a library, or that teaching yoga and meditation is pushing a form of religion. While a data-centric approach has merit, and you will find many references to the hard work of researchers recording what is happening in the growing field within these pages, this book will urge you to think about program planning and delivery from a different direction, one that aims to empower you to answer all the questions of "How?" with a resounding "Yes!" This approach is borrowed from consultant Peter Block's approach in his book *The Answer to How Is Yes: Acting on What Matters*:

> We also deny ourselves action when we keep looking for more and more information to ensure greater certainty about the future as a condition of moving on. We can turn curiosity into a life stance, in which life is to be studied, measured, submitted to a continual cost-benefit analysis, rather than lived. We can make a career of evaluating the adventures of others. The will to evaluate and measure is in the same category as the will to hold power. . . . My experience is that data and measures are not half as persuasive as anecdotes. Anecdotes, personal stories, reminiscences like biblical parables, are the medium through which faith is restored. Stories are a form of poetry, and give us a saving image to personally relate to. The persistent questions about data and evidence are most often a form of disagreement, or despair, or show a lack of faith. There is little discussion of faith in organizations, but it is only with faith that significant changes can begin.[13]

While this book will certainly answer many "How?" questions, it will do so through enthusiastic stories of what is working well elsewhere, rather than through a dry presentation of academic evidence. Ultimately the only answers that count will come from *you*—from you playing with the formats, trying out the programs for yourself, and adapting the models to what works best for your team and your community. Or for trying it and deciding it isn't for you after all. But I don't think that's going to happen. You're not so easily deterred. You're a librarian, after all.

Organization of This Book

The first two chapters of this book, "What Are Mindfulness and Meditation?" and "What Is Yoga?," will succinctly explore the very storied and complex topics of meditation, mindfulness, and yoga, so that we can make sure going forward we're all operating from the same framework of understanding. This will be the foundation on which we build everything else. We can't sell the idea of offering these types of programs in libraries to our stakeholders if we can't agree on what we're talking about and deliver that information clearly.

Chapter 3, "Implementing Yoga and Meditation Programs in Your Library," gets into the real-world issues of programming, such as marketing, planning, finding funding, and how to get buy-in from your administration. Chapter 4, "Choosing Resources and Designing Spaces," takes those plans into the spaces themselves and talks about how we carve out a niche in our existing buildings to house mindfulness programs, and where to get the supplies we need, such as yoga mats, or further training for our staff.

While on the subject of spaces and resources, chapter 5, "Passive Programs and Alternative Collections," shares sneaky—but cost- and time-effective—ways of incorporating mindfulness programs into our spaces without having to teach *any* yoga or meditation ourselves. Those who were on the fence about this—breathe a collective sigh of relief! It will also delve into alternative collections that we can circulate, and even share online, to promote wellness in our communities.

It wouldn't be a public library without someone complaining or making threats, so chapter 6, "Policies and Procedures for Avoiding and Handling Problems," is there to help answer all your "Yes. But . . ." and "What if . . ." sort of questions. It will go over liability issues, how to find reputable instructors, photo/video release waivers, consent for hands-on assists in yoga, and what to do when someone inevitably, and indignantly, informs you (sometimes in ALL CAPS on social media) that "yoga is a religion and has no business in the public library that is supported by tax dollars!"

Every chapter that follows is where we get to start having fun. This is where you are going to find program models to get you started holding yoga and meditation programs in your library. Right now. You can just open a chapter and—*bam!*—there is a tried-and-true program all ready to go, including helpful hints of what works and what doesn't. Each program tells you what you need to do in advance of the program, provides a list of needed materials, gives you a rough budget estimate of how much the program will cost, and lists in detail how to roll out the program on the day of the event. There are even handy infographics of the yoga sequences you can photocopy, or download and print, to hand out to patrons to take home for their personal practice.[14]

Each chapter also includes a list of resources for collection development, so you can help provide information to your patrons, and another list of resources for professional development so you can better educate yourself. In an effort to present all sides, I've included suggested reading that may actually refute some of this book's claims.

☉ Disclaimers, or the Fine Print

I will mention several times throughout this book that I am not a medical professional, and more than likely, neither are you. So I strongly recommend that you consult with your physician before beginning any exercise program, including yoga, and would ask you to advise your patrons to do the same. It is very important that you have them sign a liability waiver (more on this in chapter 6) stating that they agree they are voluntarily participating in movement-based activities at their own risk and that if they incur any injuries as a result of the library's programs, they will assume responsibility for it. Guardians also need to sign these on behalf of their underage children.

While all the programs presented in this book are of a secular nature, I want to make note of the fact that many of the resources that I recommend in this book and the foundations upon which yoga and meditation are built do have spiritual underpinnings. To deny that reality and pretend there are no spiritual affiliations would be dishonest, and frankly unfair to thousands of years of human history. For example, you cannot separate the commonplace adjective "zen" describing uber-laid-back behavior (as in, "Matt is like, totally zen; he didn't even get upset when his hair caught on fire") from the Japanese religion Zen. There is much overlap in today's culture between the religious and the secular, and libraries are no exception, no matter how hard we may try. The "Is yoga/meditation religious?" issue will be addressed from a practical standpoint in chapter 6, but suffice it to say that yoga is practiced in many religious traditions, and so is meditation, but that does not mean they cannot be presented in a secular fashion. I think it is important to check in with ourselves (and others) and make sure our own biases aren't dribbling over into our work too much. I don't mind sharing that I come from a diverse religious background, having been raised by two agnostic parents and a devout evangelical Pentecostal grand-mother. Sometimes I swore and wore lipstick, but on Sundays I wore dresses and combed out my long hair. My undergraduate alma mater is faith based (Baptist), and I have a minor in religious studies. I defected from the Pentecostal Church first at age thirteen, and then again in my early twenties (after a brief reunion). I then went my own way and studied multiple faiths. I finally settled into a benign agnostic Buddhism and have stayed here comfortably for over a decade. I am not neutral. Librarians are not neutral. We are human. But it is our responsibility to present all information and perspectives in a safe, honest, and respectful way. Our role as librarians is not to indoctrinate anyone with our personal religious practices or opinions, but to offer patrons information from a variety of sources and give them access to wellness tools from which they may better their lives.

⊚ You Are Part of an Important Experiment, or the Revolution

As I stated above, as librarians our mandate is to present all the available information, not just that which supports our own personal biases. Yoga, meditation, and any activity that improves physical literacy have been invaluable teaching tools in my own life and career, and in the libraries and communities where I've worked. And also in the communities I've been following in my decade of research on the topic. But—from an objective perspective—it's a relatively small sample size. This whole "does offering yoga and medi-tation at the library *really* improve people's lives?" business could honestly be considered an open-ended, long-term experiment. But I've seen strangers form lasting bonds over Down Dog. I've had depressed patrons tell me that a library's mindfulness program saved their lives. I watched an immigrant family of four cry and hold each other with gratitude after doing a group loving-kindness meditation. I've worked with young patrons with autism who couldn't communicate verbally, or grasp a pencil properly, but who could express themselves kinetically through yoga poses and free play. The definitive results of this experiment may not be in for decades. It's a risk I'm willing to take.

At some point (and this is hard for librarians!) we need to stop researching, stop looking for fail-safe directions, and just jump in with both feet. That is where our faith in the process comes in. In that spirit, I hope you'll let this book serve as inspiration for the many exciting, innovative programs you will soon deliver in your own community. Let it arm you with awareness that you too can do this. Let's get moving mindfully!

⊚ Notes

1. Lydia Saad, "Eight in 10 Americans Afflicted by Stress," Gallup, December 20, 2017, https://news.gallup.com/poll/224336/eight-americans-afflicted-stress.aspx.

2. American Psychological Association, *Stress in America: The State of our Nation*, November 1, 2017, https://www.apa.org/news/press/releases/stress/2017/state-nation.pdf.

3. Alex Therrien, "Lack of Exercise Puts One in Four People at Risk, WHO Says," BBC News, September 5, 2018, https://www.bbc.com/news/health-45408017.

4. Ann Hagell et al., "The Social Determinants of Young People's Health," *Health Foundation*, June 2018, https://www.health.org.uk/publication/social-determinants-young-peoples-health.

5. Noah Lenstra, "Let's Move in Libraries," Let's Move in Libraries, 2017, http://www.LetsMoveLibraries.org/.

6. Jenn Carson, *Physical Literacy: Movement-Based Programs in Libraries*, survey, September 8, 2017, personal author notes.

7. Lenstra, "Let's Move in Libraries."

8. Jenn Carson, *Get Your Community Moving: Physical Literacy Programs for All Ages* (Chicago: ALA Editions, 2018).

9. Tainya C. Clarke et al., "Trends in the Use of Complementary Health Approaches among Adults: United States, 2002–2012," *National Health Statistics Reports*, no 79, (Hyattsville, MD: National Center for Health Statistics, 2015), https://nccih.nih.gov/research/statistics/NHIS/2012.

10. Clarke et al., "Trends."

11. Naomi Thomas, "Yoga and Meditation on the Rise among US Adults and Kids," CNN, November 8, 2018, https://www.cnn.com/2018/11/08/health/yoga-meditation-rising-cdc-re port/index.html?fbclid=IwAR16A8c5ax0Lr4eL8qeWpcm4R04hGDIg7s1M5FFRnN4zAw 4Pv93ZNZke-TQ.

12. Linda A. Christian, "A Passion Deficit: Occupational Burnout and the New Librarian: A Recommendation Report," *Southeastern Librarian* 62, no. 4, article 2 (2016), https://digitalcom mons.kennesaw.edu/seln/vol62/iss4/2.

13. Peter Block, *The Answer to How Is Yes: Acting on What Matters* (San Francisco: Berrett-Koehler, 2001), 42–43.

14. See www.jenncarson.com.

Acknowledgments

I am a single mother of two young boys with a full-time library directorship, a busy teaching and traveling schedule, and I also write books, among other things. There is no way I could do any of this without the help of many, many people. From my neighbor Kara Pendrigh-Fowlie who walks my youngest son home from school to fellow writer Sarah Butland who sends me snail mail encouragements just when I need them—my life is full of beloveds. And while I can't possibly list all of you here, know that every smile, every cup of tea, every gentle reminder to "stop typing and get some fresh air" matters to me.

Noah Lenstra, your support of my work these last three years and your willingness to say "Yes!" to all our collaborations keeps me going when I get bogged down in bureaucracy and worried I'm not making a difference. You keep me moving (pun gleefully intended).

A big high five goes out to my boys' nanny Ebony Scott, who is also the talented photographer of many pictures in this book. She goes above and beyond the call of duty—delivering me home-cooked meals when I'm writing on a deadline, teaching the boys piano and guitar, supervising cello practice, and schlepping them over to the library to see their exhausted mom and gobble endless piles of picture books and graphic novels.

Thank you to Drew Gilbert and Karen Ruet, both friends and former colleagues from the New Brunswick College of Craft and Design, who also took photographs for this book. I am blessed to know such gifted and generous humans.

Speaking of which, this book couldn't have been written without my Sam-of-all-trades. Between climbing forty-foot ladders to repair my leaky chimney, meticulously proofreading half of this book—including the copy for the infographics—and even taking a stab at designing an infographic himself (having no previous knowledge of graphic design whatsoever), he somehow also managed to find the time (and nerve!) to be a model for an impromptu reshoot of several yoga poses a few days before deadline. While also helping me prepare for my upcoming blue belt test at Jiu Jitsu. Samuel Holmes, take a bow.

Brendan Helmuth, this is our second book together and your infographic layout just keeps getting better and better. Your photographs in this book are also incredibly valuable, as is your ongoing friendship. I love you.

Mum, what more could a daughter want than a freezer full of your homemade pies? And Janice Gagnon, your muffins are right up there, along with Ellen Helmuth's turkey dinners. I swear if love could be measured in calories, I'd never be hungry.

To my yoga and meditation students, I have learned so much from you over the years. Thank you for holding safe space with me. For sharing your stories. For trusting me as a witness on your journey to loving and cherishing your precious bodies and beings. *Namaste*.

And to Ben and Oli, my book ninjas, my mini yoga models, you are, as Karen Ruet likes to call you, "personality plus plus." My life would be so empty without you to call my home.

CHAPTER 1

What Are Mindfulness and Meditation?

IN THIS CHAPTER

▷ Defining mindfulness and meditation

▷ Determining the purpose of mindfulness and meditation programs in libraries

▷ Reviewing current mindfulness and meditation programming in libraries

---

What Is Mindfulness?

WE ARE THE WATCHER. The doer of things. And we watch ourselves while we do those things. We watch the emotions as they arise while we do them. The thoughts that may flitter past, or get stuck in tight grinding patterns. Mindfulness is that awareness. You cannot acknowledge what you are not aware of. We have a mind, yes, but we can also observe the workings of the mind, so we are therefore not "the mind." In this same way, mindfulness also impacts the way we approach our body. We have a body, yes, but we are not "the body." We do things, but we are not the things we do. We have thoughts, but we are not those thoughts. As Ajahn Chah so eloquently puts it:

> Even if your house is flooded or burnt to the ground, whatever the danger that threatens it, let it concern only the house. If there's a flood, don't let it flood your mind. If there's a fire, don't let it burn your heart. Let it be merely the house, that which is external to you, that is flooded and burned. Allow the mind to let go of its attachments. The time is ripe.[1]

He goes on to say that the body and the mind, like the house in his story, are not yours and you are not them. In the same way that your house is only yours in name, you cannot carry it around, or take it with you when you die. The same goes for the mind and the body (or your money, family, friends, possessions, etc.). Mindfulness is living your life with this approach. Anything—eating, washing dishes, crying, praying, watching TV, driving, exercising—can be done mindfully. Mindfulness, according to Susan L. Smalley and Diana Winston, "is the art of observing your physical, emotional, and mental experiences with deliberate, open and curious attention."[2] We just need to train our brains to want to go along with it. Meditation is a tool to get there.

What Is Meditation?

After you read this paragraph, take a moment and close your eyes. Rest your hands in your lap comfortably, sit up with a straight spine, and take a deep breath down into your belly. Notice how your belly moves out a little bit as your lungs fill with air, and then notice how your belly button moves back toward your spine as you let the air go. Breathe in and out, mentally observing the breath, observing the belly. Thoughts may come into your mind, and when they do say to yourself (in your head), "Thinking," and then go back to breathing. As the thoughts come back, no matter what they are, and what emotions may come with them, label them as "thinking" and then go back to focusing on your breath. Do this a few more times and then open your eyes.

There! You just experienced meditation. Simple, right? As many Zen teachers will tell you, it is the simplest thing in the world and that is why almost no one can do it. We humans seem addicted to the drama and complication of reacting. We seem to prefer it. At least on the surface. But maybe it's just because we're like fish and being reactionary is the water we grew up in. Maybe no one showed us any other way to be. We just spend our lives feeling out of control and using lots of not-so-helpful coping mechanisms (like eating disorders, alcoholism, drug addiction, shopping, social withdrawal, obsessive video game playing, etc.) to try to deal with our suffering. And we all have suffering. Eventually some people—often out of desperation—find their way to the meditation cushion to counteract all the chaos of life by focusing on something they can control: the breath.

Why Create Meditation Programs in Libraries?

You may be thinking, "Well, great. But why should libraries care?" As publicly funded institutions providing free programs, public libraries are in a unique position to offer relief from suffering to thousands, potentially millions, of people in North America and beyond. Americans visited their public libraries more than a billion times in 2015.[3] Nearly two-thirds of Canadians have a library card (about the same amount as carry passports) and visit their public libraries almost as often as they visit movie theaters.[4] With a little bit of training and the help of community volunteers or hired instructors, libraries can begin offering basic meditation programs, which have been proven to lower blood pressure and produce feelings of well-being in only fifteen minutes per day.[5] These life-changing tools can also be taught to children and teens, giving them the skills to navigate our challenging, and constantly changing, culture. We can even teach meditation to children through storytelling, as part of our existing storytime programming, or in stand-alone sessions. Children learn particularly well through mimesis and dramatic play, and we can meet multiple goals by incorporating our Every Child Ready to Read best practices into mindfulness programs.[6] Even if patrons never attend a single meditation program at the library, by providing access to quiet, contemplative spaces that are safe, warm, and dry, we are encouraging the consumption of slow information and supporting the whole person, without asking them to buy anything, or do anything for us in return.[7] That in itself is revolutionary in the fast-paced, chaotic, and politically unstable times we live in.

☺ A Look at Current Meditation Programs in Libraries

Libraries, both academic and public, are beginning to see the benefits of offering meditation programs to patrons and staff. In a 2016 survey of staff in public, academic, and school libraries, 27.8 percent of 579 respondents said their libraries offered mindfulness programs (which included breathing/walking meditation or yoga) to staff and 21 percent of 578 respondents said their libraries offered mindfulness programs to patrons.[8] That's a significant amount!

Meditation and mindfulness-based stress reduction programs are also popping up in North American prisons. Meditation books and audiobooks are being made available through prison libraries.[9] Dr. Drew Leder, a leading expert on wellness programs in prisons and a regular prison volunteer, believes meditation helps inmates in three important ways: by lowering the inmates' reactivity and impulsivity, by helping them develop a deep spiritual practice that gives their lives meaning, and by helping them feel calm in a toxic environment.[10] Leder stresses the importance of working closely with prison librarians to provide meditation, and if there is no space or opportunity available to run a program to still provide resources in the form of pamphlets, books, audiobooks, and online courses. The Prison Mindfulness Institute maintains a list of programs being offered through US prisons. If you are a prison librarian, be sure to visit its website for instructions on how to offer meditation and mindfulness resources in your prison library.[11]

So whether you work in a public or private library setting—in a hospital, archive, prison, or corporate office—know that you are not alone in wishing to bring the benefits of meditation to your patrons. While this book focuses mostly on offering meditation and mindfulness sessions in public, academic, and school libraries, know that any of these program models could easily be adapted to meet the needs of your patrons in your particular environment. All you need is a little creativity and (hopefully) a cooperative administration.

☺ Key Points

- Mindfulness is the deliberate observation of your thoughts, emotions, actions, and surroundings.
- Meditation is the deliberate act of sitting or moving in a mindful manner while observing the breath or thoughts with the intention of obtaining an inner quietening.
- Libraries—as community centers with little to no barriers to entry or access of services—are perfectly poised to offer mindfulness tools (such as meditation training) and materials (like books), or to simply provide spaces for contemplation, to as many people as possible.
- Public, academic, prison, and other libraries are already offering meditation services, and the trend continues to grow.

☺ Notes

1. Ajahn Chah, "Advice for Someone Who Is Dying," *Lion's Roar*, October 26, 2018, https://www.lionsroar.com/our-real-home-death/.

2. Susan L. Smalley and Diana Winston, *Fully Present: The Science, Art, and Practice of Mindfulness* (New York: Da Capo Lifelong Books, 2010).

3. Elizabeth Holton, "People Visited Public Libraries More Than a Billion Times in 2015," Institute of Museum and Library Services, August 2, 2018, https://www.imls.gov/news-events/news-releases/people-visited-public-libraries-more-billion-times-2015.

4. Online Computer Library Center (OCLC), *How Canadian Public Libraries Stack Up*, Online Computer Library Center, 2012, https://www.oclc.org/content/dam/oclc/reports/canadastackup/214109cef_how_libraries_stack_up.pdf.

5. OCLC, *How Canadian Public Libraries Stack Up*.

6. American Library Association (ALA), *Every Child Ready to Read @ Your Library*, accessed November 10, 2018, http://everychildreadytoread.org/.

7. Oleg Kagan, "Slow Info: Where Libraries, Reading, and Well-Being Converge," *EveryLibrary* (blog), January 23, 2018, https://medium.com/everylibrary/slow-info-where-libraries-reading-and-well-being-converge-44de619df0b8.

8. Richard Moniz et al., *Mindfulness Survey* (2016), obtained through private email correspondence with Richard Moniz, July 12, 2018.

9. Thomas Lyons and William Dustin Cantrell, "Prison Meditation Movements and Mass Incarceration," *International Journal of Offender Therapy and Comparative Criminology* 60, no. 12 (2016): 1363–75, https://www.ncbi.nlm.nih.gov/pmc/articles/PMC4633398/.

10. Jails to Jobs, "How Practicing Meditation in Prison Can Help Inmates Cope," *Jails to Jobs* (blog), January 12, 2017, https://www.jailstojobs.org/how-practicing-meditation-in-prison-can-help-inmates-cope/.

11. Prison Mindfulness Institute, "Books behind Bars," Prison Mindfulness Institute, accessed November 1, 2018, https://www.prisonmindfulness.org/projects/books-behind-bars/.

CHAPTER 2

What Is Yoga?

IN THIS CHAPTER

▷ Defining yoga

▷ Determining the purpose of yoga programs in libraries

▷ Reviewing current yoga programming in libraries

What Is Yoga?

EVERYWHERE YOU LOOK there are people doing yoga: on the cover of *Yoga Journal*, at the airport, on that famous clothing company's billboard, on reality TV, and probably in your neighborhood (or even your local library!). But what *is* yoga, exactly? The word "yoga" means "union," to yoke, to join together. Yoga is the joining of the mind, spirit, and body to bring the whole person into harmony. It is an eight-limbed system designed to lead a person toward enlightenment, of which *Hatha* yoga (the physical poses we see all those people in stretchy pants doing) is only one component. The physical poses are designed to calm and focus the mind while preparing the body for long periods of contemplation and meditation. Some consider it to be a form of embodied mindfulness, a moving form of meditation.[1] Yoga as a philosophical system has been around for an estimated five thousand years, but many of the poses have only been added over the last few centuries. *Hatha* yoga isn't a religion or a cult, so there are no worries about indoctrinating any of your patrons or students, but yoga, like meditation, *is* practiced by people of all different religions and cultures, which makes offering it at the library a great opportunity to bring people from various communities together.

There has been an explosion of different types of yoga in the West in the last thirty years as teachers and moneymakers scramble to trademark their own personal brand of yoga and profit from its current trendiness. There has been much controversy over whether yoga poses or sequences can be considered a teacher's "original work," and therefore subject to copyright law or patent law, and the final ruling in this matter was "No."[2] If you'd like to know more about the different styles of *Hatha* yoga before you start looking for an instructor or training program, consult Meagan McCrary's book *Pick Your Yoga Practice: Exploring and Understanding Different Styles of Yoga.*[3]

Why Create Yoga Programs in Libraries?

As discussed in the previous chapter, meditation (and remember, yoga is a moving form of meditation) has been proven to lower blood pressure and lead to a greater sense of well-being. If you read some of the alarming statistics in the preface of this book, you will want to know everything you can about how to avert our current health crisis. Yoga is one of the ways we can do that. According to the American Osteopathic Association, yoga can increase flexibility and muscle tone, improve cardiovascular and respiratory health, improve athletic performance, and help maintain a healthy weight.[4] Yoga has even been proven to reduce the symptoms of depression and chronic back pain.[5] In a world teeming with messages about how we have to go faster, buy more, look perfect, and hustle, hustle, hustle, libraries and librarians are perfectly poised as, what Thomas Moore calls, "inefficiency experts" to offer some slow information.[6]

Libraries invite people to slow down, pick up a book or newspaper, sit in the sunshine and sip some coffee, attend an author's talk, and yes, even join a yoga class. Ben Katt, well-known pastor and podcast host, confessed in an essay titled "The Art of Being Inefficient" that he gave up running in order to start practicing yoga on his lunch break.[7] With three kids, a wife, an online following, a large congregation, and a non-profit to manage, he felt he was doing good work, but also felt like he wasn't *enjoying* any of it. I'm sure the over-worked and overwhelmed librarians reading this right now can relate. He was determined to be less outcome focused, at least in his downtime: "It was the least efficient thing I could have done—to move slowly and then be still on a mat for an hour in the middle of the day when I could have scheduled a lunch meeting or caught up on a project."[8] What if libraries could be that safe, quiet space people come to on their lunch break to stretch out on the mat? In some places, like my library in Woodstock, New Brunswick, Canada, we already are. And we're not the only ones.

Current Yoga Programs in Libraries

Over the past decade I have held more yoga programs in libraries, schools, community centers, conference halls, day cares, and parks than I can count. I've even taught yoga online in webinars or through YouTube videos. I've made yoga sequences into handouts and given them to people to take home to practice on their own. My small-town public library has offered Mom & Baby Yoga, Rhythm & Flow Yoga (with live music), Yoga for Heartache, Yoga for Trauma, Yoga for Runners, Yoga for Walkers, Chair Yoga, Laughter Yoga, Gentle Yoga, Yoga for Stress Relief, Yoga for Gardeners, Yoga for Teens, Family Yoga Parties, Yoga for Knitters, and so much more. I knew I couldn't be the only yogi-librarian who was easily attracting fifteen to twenty-plus people to yoga classes every week.

When I created a survey in the spring of 2017 that was administered through the American Library Association's member newsletter, of the more than three hundred librarians who responded, 65 percent said they offered some form of programming that encouraged physical activity.[9] The majority of those activities were yoga classes. That same spring, I helped Dr. Noah Lenstra design a survey that was responded to by more than sixteen hundred library staff across North America. The majority of respondents, just like with my survey, were from public, school, or academic libraries. Lenstra provided a list of movement-based programs and asked respondents to indicate which had been offered at their libraries (either currently, or in the recent past).[10] Can you guess what the most popular answer was? Yoga. By 65 percent of respondents. That seems to be pretty solid evidence that if you walk into three public, academic, or school libraries this week, at least two of them have probably offered a physical literacy program at some point, and it was most likely a yoga class. And if not, maybe they will tomorrow. Especially if you leave them a copy of this book.

⑨ Key Points

- Yoga is a moving form of meditation that facilitates the joining of the mind, spirit, and body to bring the whole person into a state of cohesion, which promotes wellness and lowers stress levels.
- Yoga has been proven to improve mental and physical health in controlled trials.
- Libraries—as existing "inefficiency experts" and safe, accessible community centers—are perfectly poised to offer yoga to as many people as possible.
- According to recent surveys, 65 percent of public, school, and academic libraries have already offered a yoga class at some point, and the trend continues to grow.

⑨ Notes

1. Cyndi Lee, "How to Practice Embodied Mindfulness," *Lion's Roar*, April 28, 2017, https://www.lionsroar.com/how-to-practice-embodied-mindfulness/?utm_content=bufferdda4b&utm_medium=social&utm_source=facebook.com&utm_campaign=buffer.

2. Anandashankar Mazumdar, "The Bikram Lawsuits and Why It Matters to You," Yoga Alliance, April 18, 2013, https://www.yogaalliance.org/Learn/Articles/bikram_lawsuits_4_18_2013.

3. Meagan McCrary, *Pick Your Yoga Practice: Exploring and Understanding Different Styles of Yoga* (San Francisco: New World Library, 2013).

4. American Osteopathic Association, "Maintaining a Regular Yoga Practice Can Provide Physical and Mental Health Benefits," *The Benefits of Yoga*, accessed November 13, 2018, https://osteopathic.org/what-is-osteopathic-medicine/benefits-of-yoga/.

5. Amanda MacMillan, "It's Official: Yoga Helps Depression," *Time*, March 8, 2017, http://time.com/4695558/yoga-breathing-depression/; Amanda MacMillan, "Yoga May Be Good for Stubborn Back Pain," *Time*, January 12, 2017, http://time.com/4632204/yoga-lower-back-pain/?iid=sr-link6.

6. Thomas Moore, *The Re-enchantment of Everyday Life* (New York: Harper Perennial, 1997).

7. Ben Katt, "The Art of Being Inefficient," *On Being Blog*, April 9, 2018, https://onbeing.org/blog/ben-katt-the-art-of-being-inefficient/.

8. Katt, "Art of Being Inefficient."

9. Jenn Carson, *Physical Literacy: Movement-Based Programs in Libraries*, survey, September 8, 2017, personal author notes.

10. Noah Lenstra, "Movement-Based Programs in U.S. and Canadian Public Libraries: Evidence of Impacts from an Exploratory Survey," *Evidence Based Library and Information Practice* 12, no. 4 (2017): 214–32.

CHAPTER 3

Implementing Yoga and Meditation Programs in Your Library

IN THIS CHAPTER

▷ Garnering support from your stakeholders

▷ Identifying your audience

▷ Identifying who will teach your program

▷ Training required for program delivery

▷ Logistics: dates/times/locations

▷ Funding your program

▷ Working with community partners

▷ Marketing your program

▷ Evaluating yoga and meditation programs

Getting Support from Your Stakeholders

THIS CHAPTER AND CHAPTER 6, "Policies and Procedures for Avoiding and Handling Problems," are designed to help answer the many conflicting questions you are bound to get from your administration, board members, volunteers, staff, and patrons (and perhaps even the media) when announcing you'd like to start teaching yoga and meditation at the library. For one, these two things may seem to be in opposition: Aren't yoga classes full of loud music and aren't libraries supposed to be quiet like Zen monasteries? Don't meditation and yoga have religious roots? What if someone gets hurt? Wait, where are we going to find the time and money for this?!

Fear not, by the end of this book most of these questions should be answered, or at least on their way to being answered. Read these chapters; highlight and photocopy the most pressing concerns brought about by your board or staff, and present them with the answers from someone who has done it before. I've made mistakes, tried out programs that flopped, and took risks so that you could walk forward with confidence knowing what works and what doesn't and be willing to take a few risks of your own. Let's get started!

Identifying Your Audience

Once you decide you would like to try offering a yoga or meditation program in your library, then you have to think about whom you would most like to deliver the program to. It's best to ask yourself these sorts of questions:

- What need am I trying to fill in my community?
- Who would most benefit from this program?
- Who would be most receptive to this program?

Being very clear about the purpose of your program will help you to zero in on your target audience and then later help figure out how to market to them. For example, let's say you wanted to offer a Chair Yoga program because you thought it sounded like something you felt comfortable teaching. You would need to determine if children were allowed to attend, or if you'd only offer it to adults, or if you'd like to market it directly to seniors. Who might need or want Chair Yoga the most? Who might actually show up?

Another example might be a Yoga for Heartache class. How do you determine who has heartache? Well, you can't. Plus, the nature of some of the discussion in class among the students might not be suitable for certain ages, so you may need to make the program adults only. But children have heartache too. Could you make a special class just for them? What about if your library is in a high school? A grief-focused yoga session for certain teens might be highly appropriate. You could enlist your high school's guidance counselor (or psychologist, if you have one) to recommend students for the program and act in an advisory role.

The program models in this book are divided by age demographics, but almost all the programs could be easily adapted to different groups, and suggestions are made to help facilitate this in each chapter. If you have access to a recent community needs assessment, that is a good place to start looking for answers to the important question of whom we should be programming for in your library.

Who Will Teach Your Program?

Once you've decided what sort of program you are going to run and who is going to attend, then you need to determine who will lead the session. Do you presently have a staff member who has yoga or meditation training, or even experience or interest? Would that staff member be willing to take some training? Are you? Is there funding available for that?

Do you have volunteers that would be keen to help? Do you have any friends or family members who happen to be yoga teachers or regular meditators? What about approaching local yoga studios or meditation halls to recruit possible volunteers (or paid instructors)? You could even put a call out on social media asking if anyone has experience with these subjects to contact the library. This could give you a built-in audience and possible teacher contacts. If you are holding a very specific kind of class, such as a trauma-informed yoga program, you're going to need to seek out someone with specialized training.

When I hire library staff I look to see what secondary skills they have—besides a good customer service/library background, of course!—and ask them if they would be happy to use these skills in their new workplace. Because of this technique, I've recruited two professional photographers/videographers, a graphic designer, and a musician. Perhaps you can find a yoga teacher/summer student or meditating IT guru?

Training Required for Teaching Yoga and Meditation

There is presently no governing body for yoga or meditation instruction. While member groups, such as Yoga Alliance and the International Association of Yoga Therapists, exist and have attempted to provide requirements for teacher training programs, there's nothing to stop anyone with a pair of stretchy pants or a meditation cushion from hanging out a shingle (or in modern-day vernacular, creating a website) and calling themselves a "teacher." So what do you look for when searching for a teacher at your library, or researching training for yourself or staff? The baseline standard for beginner yoga teachers is a two-hundred-hour training program in *Hatha* yoga (the physical component), though most teacher trainings will touch on all eight branches of yoga, including *Pranayama* (breath work) and meditation. Five hundred hours is considered an advanced level of certification. Additional hours may be added to specialize in certain disciplines, such as Aerial Yoga (done suspended in hammocks like Cirque de Soleil performers), Chair Yoga, or Yin (poses are held longer, usually three to five minutes to help connective tissue release). Many teachers are also taking complementary courses, such as sports-medicine-style self-massage (using foam rollers and lacrosse balls), Thai Therapeutic Massage (partner massage done by manipulating each other's limbs) or Yoga *Nidra* (guided sleeplike meditation done lying down) in order to offer more comprehensive services to their clients. Others combine their career practices in disciplines such as physiotherapy, social work, chiropractic care, psychology, or nursing with yoga teaching and undertake certification to become yoga therapists, which applies yoga in a clinical setting for specific health issues, such as arthritis, trauma recovery, drug addiction, and cancer. When searching out an instructor, inquire as to their training and certifications, and ask to see copies of their diplomas. You should also ask for references, like you would for any other volunteer or staff member. Make sure to have them provide a criminal record check in order to work with the vulnerable sector (children, disabled, and the elderly), if that is available in your municipality. You can check with your library's insurance policy, but many policies only cover the staff and public participating in library programs, not outside instructors (paid or otherwise). In either case, it is always a good idea to request that your instructors have proof of personal liability insurance. If you are looking into purchasing it for yourself, it is about $200 annually.

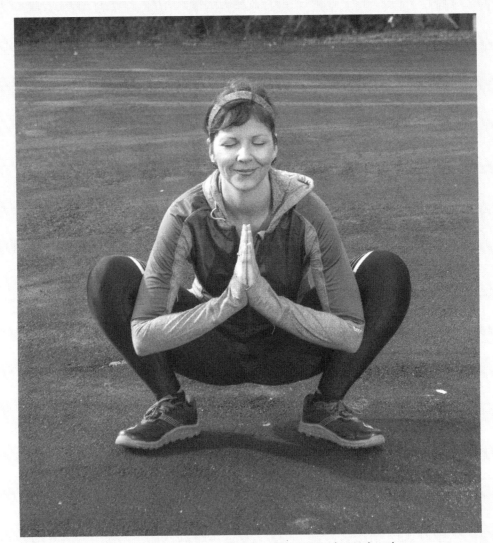

Figure 3.1. Take a moment to yourself before class. *Brendan Helmuth*

A word of advice for yoga/meditation teacher–librarians: make sure before you begin any mindfulness-based program to take a moment or two to center yourself. Allow yourself a few minutes to sit quietly and follow your breath, take a gentle stroll around the block, or have a cup of tea in the break room. If you rush into class harried and overwhelmed, your students will feed off that energy. Instead, if you come in relaxed and with clear intention to create safe space, they will feel nurtured, calm, and welcome. Remember, for many of them, this is the first time trying yoga or meditation, and they may be experiencing a lot of anxiety or hesitation. Likewise, be gentle with yourself. If you are going through a personal or work-related crisis; are sick, irritable, approaching burnout; and are having your own difficulties staying present, it may be best to turn the class over to another teacher temporarily. Yoga and meditation can be a wonderful tool for helping deal with difficult emotions and life circumstances, and we have to model the behavior we teach about in class: being gentle, patient, and persistently loving with ourselves.

◎ Logistics: Dates/Times/Locations

You may be wondering about the logistics of this sort of programming. Where and when to host yoga and meditation classes are entirely dependent on the audience and subject of the session in question. The next chapter will explore what sort of spaces are appropriate for teaching yoga and meditation. Each program model in the programming chapters will discuss the best time of day to host that particular event, as well as the space, staff/volunteers, and props required. Keep reading!

◎ Paying for Your Program

You may also be wondering what sort of cost is involved in teaching yoga and meditation. I'm not going to lie to you: yoga mats aren't cheap, especially when you are ordering twenty-plus of them. Bolsters are even worse (which is why I don't have any—yet!). Setting yourself up to teach yoga at the library for the first time is not going to be easy on your budget. But the good news is that once you buy the most basic props (more on what these are and where to get them in the next chapter), the rest of your programs aren't going to cost you much of anything. Yes, it is a big initial investment, but it will pay off for years! And remember, there are *always* work-arounds. Find instructors who can bring their own props with them. Ask students to provide their own mats. Hold a yoga program on the storytime carpet. Do meditation using the existing desk chairs. Have a sewing night at the library and make some eye pillows and beanbags with donated fabric scraps. You are only limited by your own imagination.

I'm sure my staff sometimes wonder what I'm doing in my office all day, buried in piles of paper. I'm usually applying for grants. My provincially and municipally funded public library doesn't have a very large programming budget, so in order for us to be able to offer as many programs as we do (630 programs in 2017!), I'm entirely dependent on outside funding sources. Start thinking about researching wellness grants, healthy living grants, mental health grants, food security grants, physical literacy grants, literacy grants, indigenous services grants, and many others. You can even apply directly for yoga grants through the Give Back Yoga Foundation.[1] Look to see what is available in your area and start applying. People won't give you money if you don't ask. Also consider working with your Friends group to fund-raise to support your new yoga and meditation programs. You could make a poster with a giant rolled-up yoga mat drawn on it and color up the mat in increments until you reach the top (and your goal). Think outside the box!

◎ Using Community Partners

Sometimes we get lucky and the people or organizations we partner with also provide us with the monetary funds or materials required to run our program successfully. It could be something simple, like you want to have a mindful eating program where you peel oranges and eat them slowly, but you have no oranges and no money to buy them. But you can call or visit a local farmer, grocer, market, or distributer to see if they would donate some. Offer to put their logo on the poster and Facebook event and give them a big shout-out to everyone who attends.

Sometimes you can establish deeper, ongoing kinds of collaboration. For example, we have a local Brazilian Jiu Jitsu Club in our town and a few times a year they come and give free demos or teach self-defense workshops at our library. Sometimes, if I can find some grant funding, I'll pay them a small honorarium, but even if I can't they will still bring their mats over and have a great time because it is good exposure for their club and they love sharing their sport. In exchange, once a month I bring the library's yoga mats over to their club, drop off some library event calendars, talk about our yoga programs, and give them a yoga class. I do this on my own time, because their club is only open in the evenings and Sundays (when the library isn't), but I know it is worth it, because I'm making deep community connections. And now my boys and I practice Jiu Jitsu. We also have many of the students from the club, especially the young ones, come to the library for other programs, such as Chess Club or Family Board Game Night. The instructors at the club give me advice when I'm doing collection development, offering suggestions about what martial arts books and movies to buy for the library. In partnerships like this everyone wins. Our partnership with this local sports club is just one example of how reaching out to create partnerships in your community can lead to innovative program development and delivery; for more examples, please read my first library programming book, *Get Your Community Moving: Physical Literacy Programs for All Ages*.[2]

I suggest you walk or drive over to your local meditation center and ask what sort of services they provide. They may give you all kinds of ideas for possible programs. They may be thrilled with the possibility of a larger audience being interested in meditation. They may dig out their calendars right then and ask when they can come over to the library to teach a meditation class. Remember, most people who are passionate about their hobbies or vocations are also passionate about sharing them with others. I can tell you from experience that not every attempt at creating a partnership will be successful, for myriad reasons, but I challenge you to keep trying, to keep reaching out. I *can* promise you the effort will be worth it.

Marketing Your Program

In each program model there will be suggestions for how to best market that specific event. You probably already know how to reach your local audience, but this might give you some new ideas. At my library we use Facebook events and posts, our website, print posters, print calendars, word of mouth, press releases to news outlets, and occasionally, public service announcement call-ins to radio stations. We're working on an electronic newsletter, but have to be careful of the delivery method due to the new anti-spam legislation in Canada.[3] At one time you could just take people's emails and send out newsletters or announcements, but we can't do that anymore without following a certain protocol. You might also want to consider marketing through Twitter, Instagram, paid ads, or other outlets. In my semi-rural community, Facebook, the website, a calendar, posters on bulletin boards, and word of mouth seem to work best.

Which languages are most commonly spoken in your community? Our branch sends out most of its marketing material in English since that is the mother tongue of the majority of our residents in this part of the county, but we are a bilingual (French and English) province. So all of our event information is translated into French and English for our website, so there is always at least one multilingual source. We also occasionally offer bilingual programs, and try to always have a staff member available to speak both official languages if someone requests a translation. Think about your community, review its most recent census, and decide what languages would reach the most patrons—it might be worth your while to translate these announcements in order to reach a larger audience. For larger events, consider having someone on hand to provide sign language interpretation as well, if applicable.

◎ Evaluating Your Program

Once you hold your first yoga or meditation program, how can you tell if it was a success and if you should do it again? Not only is it important to elicit feedback from your patrons, it is equally important to actually *listen* to what they have to say. Don't hand out evaluation forms if no one is going to read them or do anything about them anyway. This will breed mistrust among your clientele. It is so important to solicit feedback from a broad selection of the population, because as you already know, the patrons with especially *strong opinions* will tell you everything they are thinking anyway, whether it is valuable information or not. Listen, smile, nod, take notes, thank them for sharing, and try not to get your back up. But remember that no particular patron is more important than any other (despite what they may tell you), and it is our job to make sure we are meeting as many possible needs as we can with the skills, resources, space, and time we have, based on our organization's mission and strategic plan. So it is essential to seek feedback from the patrons who never say anything at all.

This is where evaluation forms can prove to be very helpful.[4] Hand them out at the end of a program, or else create a general survey to give out to your patrons, perhaps at your annual general meeting, asking what they would like to have offered in the year ahead. Links to digital surveys that you can share on social media are great too. There is lots of free online survey software available, like SurveyMonkey, for you to take advantage of. Especially don't forget to also solicit the opinions of the marginalized and the illiterate, who may not attend your current programs, feel comfortable with paper or electronic forms, or engage socially with the staff. Their thoughts about services are just as important. Take a moment for engagement when you are doing outreach, by asking people what they'd like to see more of at the library, or if they ever thought about trying meditation or yoga. And lastly, don't forget to gather feedback from staff, especially if you are also delivering inreach programs to them (more about that in chapter 11).

◎ Key Points

- We can garner support from stakeholders by showing them that there is strong evidence for the mental and physical health benefits of yoga and meditation, and that we can create clear policies and procedures to govern programming.
- We can identify our audience for yoga and meditation programs by asking a variety of questions about our community's needs and wants.
- We need to identify which staff member, volunteer, or community partner will deliver the program(s) most effectively.
- We need to make sure that the facilitator has the proper training required for program delivery.

- We need to determine the dates, times, and location of the programs based on the subject of each program and its audience.
- We can find funding for our programming by being creative, applying for grants, and being willing to make a large initial investment knowing it has positive long-term outcomes.
- We can work closely with community partners for sponsorship and collaborative program delivery.
- We can be creative about marketing our program(s) in ways that will reach the widest possible audience.
- Evaluating yoga and meditation programs by seeking feedback from our patrons, staff, and the general public helps us improve program delivery.

Notes

1. Give Back Yoga Foundation, "Grant Information," Give Back Yoga Foundation, accessed November 14, 2018, https://givebackyoga.org/about-our-non-profit-yoga-organization/grant-information/.

2. Jenn Carson, *Get Your Community Moving: Physical Literacy Programs for All Ages* (Chicago: ALA Editions, 2018).

3. Government of Canada, "Canada's Law on Spam and Other Electronic Threats," Canada's Anti-Spam Legislation, 2017, http://fightspam.gc.ca/eic/site/030.nsf/eng/home.

4. You can find a sample program evaluation form from my library service here: Government of New Brunswick, "Appendix B: Sample Program Evaluation Form," *The New Brunswick Public Library Service Policy 1085*, July 2017, http://www2.gnb.ca/content/dam/gnb/Departments/nbpl-sbpnb/pdf/politiques-policies/1085_library-programs_appendix-b.pdf.

Choosing Resources and Designing Spaces

Yoga and Meditation Supplies

WHEN IT COMES TO BUYING yoga and meditation supplies for your library, you need to ask yourself some important questions first:

- What types of programs do I plan to have?
- What is my audience?
- What is the budget?
- Is there an opportunity to add to resources next year and the year after, thereby growing the collection slowly?
- If so, what are the most essential tools we need now?
- What are nice extras we could add later?
- How many people do we expect to have at each program?
- How much storage space do we have?

Let me tell you right now that you can, for all intents and purposes, hold a yoga program at your library tomorrow with no supplies purchased. I'm sure somewhere in your library you have access to some folding or desk-type chairs. Ta-da! You have everything you need for a basic Chair Yoga program or Introduction to Meditation workshop. Have a large carpet you do storytime on? Perfect, you can now host a kids' yoga class. If you want to have a class where you use yoga mats, you can always ask patrons to supply their own. So stop using "But we don't have any money!!" as an excuse not to offer awesome programming. Some of my best programs over the years have cost nothing but time. But, if you have money to spend, check out the table below for a list of what you could spend it on—divided into "basic" and "fun extra" categories—with rough estimates of the cost per unit. I've listed the sizes I recommend as well. In general, if you buy in larger quantities you can get items for a cheaper price.

Table 4.1. Tools for Yoga Classes

BASIC	FUN EXTRA
Yoga mat ($15–$20)	Cotton blanket ($28)
4" foam block ($15)	24" rectangular bolster* ($50)
8' cotton strap ($15)	8' thick cylindrical bolster* ($50)
Small singing bowl ($30)	Eye pillows/beanbags* ($10)

*indicates it should be purchased with a washable cover

When purchasing mats, investing a little more into a higher-quality version means they will probably last longer. I really like Halfmoon's 4 mm Essential Studio Mats. I've been using them twice weekly (or more) at the library for three years and they look like new. At home I use the B MAT brand, which is thicker and more expensive. It also shows dirt more easily. I use B MAT Traveller for teaching on the road. B MAT also makes a B MAT Mini for kids, but they are $52 retail.

Blankets should always be cotton. Or at least a cotton-poly blend. Many people are allergic to wool (plus it is scratchy), and fleece pills and collects lint and hair. Cotton is easy to wash and only shrinks about a quarter of an inch. Meditation cushions, eye pillows/beanbags, and yoga bolsters should always have washable cotton covers.

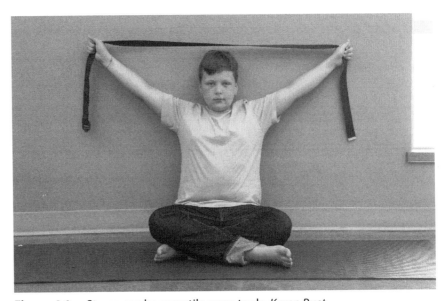

Figure 4.1. Straps can be versatile yoga tools. *Karen Ruet*

Straps should be eight feet or longer to accommodate larger bodies and more varied usage. Six-foot straps will do, but some people may have to tie two straps together, which could make them feel singled out and uncomfortable. I have six-foot straps at the library and I regret it. I bought eight-foot ones for my home studio, and they are much more accommodating.

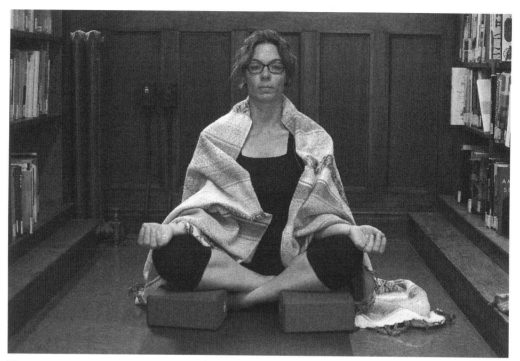

Figure 4.2. Cotton blankets and 4" blocks offer good support. *Ebony Scott*

The best blocks are four inches thick. Foam is the cheapest and lightest option (which is important if you are planning on doing outreach and will be lugging props around). I use foam blocks at the library and they are great. But they do mark easily, so ours are covered in scratches and fingernail indents (and bite marks from kids). At my home studio I have cork blocks, which are much heavier and more expensive, but much more durable. They are also steadier when using them for balancing poses. There are thinner blocks on the market, such as two-inch chip foam or three-inch foam, and it is nice to have a variety for making adjustments, but if you can only afford one set, go for the four-inch ones.

Beanbags might be something you already have kicking around your storytime props. If not, you can make them easily, or buy them cheaply through an educational supply store. My kids helped make about ten of mine, and the rest were made and donated by a yoga student and her kids.

Table 4.2. Tools for Meditation Classes

BASIC	FUN EXTRA
• Zabuton cushion* ($60)	• Meditation floor chair* ($50)
• Small singing bowl ($30)	• Zafu cushion* ($60)
• Cotton blanket ($28)	• Wooden meditation stool ($70)

*indicates it should be purchased with a washable cover

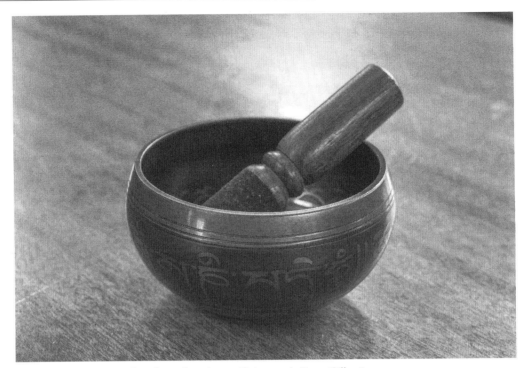

Figure 4.3. Singing bowls make a beautiful sound. *Drew Gilbert*

Most of the items can be ordered wholesale over the internet. I do recommend purchasing a singing bowl in person, so you can test out its tone. You can strike the bowl with a mallet and then rub the mallet along the edge in a circular fashion to make it "sing." These bowls can be found at yoga and meditation supply stores, Buddhist bookstores, and new age gift shops. Some stores give a wholesale discount to certified yoga teachers buying in bulk. Before placing an order, it's always a good idea to inquire and apply for their discount if you are eligible. I order all my supplies for the library online from Canadian company Halfmoon, which gives me a generous wholesale discount. Shipping is free over a certain amount, and the quality is excellent. But I've also bought products for my home studio at other locations. Here is a list of retailers I recommend based on the quality of their products and service. I am not endorsed by any of them.

- B MAT (US/Can/EU) https://byoganow.com/
- Chattra (US) https://chattra.com/
- Gaiam (US) https://www.gaiam.com/
- Halfmoon (US/Can) https://www.shophalfmoon.com/
- Manduka (US/EU) https://www.manduka.com/

⊚ How and Where to Store Your Supplies

Depending on the size of your library, your available storage space, and the types of programs you are offering, you may have to get creative about storing your yoga and meditation supplies. If you have no extra room to spare, one efficient option is recruiting yoga or meditation instructors who supply their own mats and props. As I've mentioned previously, you can also ask participants to bring their own mats, blankets, or cushions. Another option is offering programs that don't require any special equipment. Yoga and meditation can easily be done on wooden or folding chairs, which most libraries already possess. A children's yoga program can be done in the same place you deliver storytime, right on the circle carpet in the children's department, or outdoors on the lawn or in the park. Standing yoga poses can be done anywhere, even a classroom full of desks. Walking meditation can be done in a hallway, in a parking lot, or throughout the stacks.

That said, if you do go all in and buy mats, bolsters, zafus, and a singing bowl, you're going to need a place to store them. An ideal situation would be having a large storage closet that could be lined with large shelving units. The closet would be welcoming, well lit, and handy to the room where you will be hosting the programs so patrons can freely access the materials as needed, but secure enough to prevent theft. Even a large, locking storage cabinet would be swell. Or, if you wanted to make supplies like mats and cushions available to patrons to use on their own, a nice deep bookshelf in a quiet corner would do the trick.

My library's situation is less than ideal. We have an old wonky book truck with a perpetually squeaky wheel and chipped orange paint that we store the mats on. We keep the foam blocks in two cracked plastic book bins (one with a broken handle). We store the beanbags and straps in re-used bags. It isn't a classy setup, but it was free and it works.

Caring for Supplies

As mentioned previously, it is always a good idea to buy blankets that are washable and bolsters, cushions, and other supplies with washable covers. This is a library after all. People are going to get germs all over everything. Cotton straps can also be thrown in the washing machine and hung to dry. I wash everything as often as necessary, depending on how much it is used. Foam blocks and mats can be hosed off in warm weather and put out in the sun to dry. Just don't leave them too long or the color will fade. And don't leave them unattended, or they may get stolen or vandalized. Mats can also be wiped down after every class with a solution of equal parts water and white vinegar (which is a little smelly until it evaporates) or water and a couple of drops of tea tree oil in a spray bottle. Vinegar and tea tree oil contain antibacterial and anti-fungal properties that kill most of the nastiness that may be on the mats. You can use a soft cloth to do this, or paper towel. I've also used baby wipes to clean mats; just make sure they are the fragrance-and-alcohol-free kind.

Digital Resources for Yoga and Meditation

During yoga and meditation programs you are going to want to recommend all the awesome books you have available for students to check out with their library cards. I hope you've even made a great display to refer them to! You'll find a list of suggestions for collection development at the end of all the programming chapters in this book. But let's not forget about other resources that patrons might like to get their eyeballs and ears on: websites, movies, apps, and podcasts. There are a number of really useful digital resources available. Some of them, like the meditation and sleep aid Calm, which was voted as the 2017 App of the Year, have a cost associated with them (US$4.99/month for a yearly subscription), but they often have a free trial so patrons can test them out. Here are some of my favorites:

Blogs/Websites/Online Magazines

- *Elephant Journal*—https://www.elephantjournal.com/
- *Greater Good: Science-Based Insights for a Meaningful Life*—https://greatergood.berkeley.edu/
- *The Kids Yoga Resource*—http://www.thekidsyogaresource.com/
- *Lion's Roar: Buddhist Wisdom for Our Time*—https://www.lionsroar.com/
- *Mindful: Healthy Mind, Healthy Life*—https://www.mindful.org/
- *The On Being Blog*—https://onbeing.org/blog/
- *Tricycle: The Buddhist Review*—https://tricycle.org/
- Yoga in the Library—www.yogainthelibrary.com

Free Applications (for iOS and Android)

- Aura—https://www.aurahealth.io/
- Insight Timer—https://insighttimer.com/
- Stop, Breathe, Think—https://www.stopbreathethink.com/

Podcasts

- *Hello Humans*—http://hellohumans.co/
- *The One You Feed*—http://www.oneyoufeed.net/
- *Waking Up*—https://samharris.org/podcast/

Online Videos

- "A Simple Way to Break a Bad Habit" by Judson Brewer—https://www.ted.com/talks/judson_brewer_a_simple_way_to_break_a_bad_habit
- "All It Takes Is 10 Mindful Minutes" by Andy Puddicombe—https://www.ted.com/talks/andy_puddicombe_all_it_takes_is_10_mindful_minutes
- "Meditation 101: A Beginner's Guide" by Happify—https://www.youtube.com/watch?v=o-kMJBWk9E0
- "Mindfulness Animated in 3 Minutes" by AnimateEducate—https://www.youtube.com/watch?v=mjtfyuTTQFY
- "Self-Transformation through Mindfulness" by Dr. David Vago—https://www.youtube.com/watch?v=1nP5oedmzkM
- "Why Mindfulness Is a Superpower: An Animation" by Happify—https://www.youtube.com/watch?v=w6T02g5hnT4

DVDs

There are a lot of really good yoga DVDs on the market, and some pretty terrible ones. Since they can be pricey, here's a list of some of my favorites with a short review to help you decide which to purchase.

- *A.M. & P.M. Yoga for Beginners* by Rodney Yee, Colleen Saidman, and Patricia Walden.
  Bampton, ON: Gaiam, 2013. ISBN 978-0766-25651-4; US$16.98.

This is the first DVD I grab off the shelf every time someone comes into the library and says that they'd like to try yoga at home before coming to class, or that they are a beginner and would like to start a home practice. Broken into short, manageable chunks (twenty minutes each) of either energizing or relaxing classes, and also including five-minute meditations, this is the perfect resource for everyone wanting to try out yoga or meditation without making a big time commitment. The DVD is so well priced, I recommend buying two copies for when one gets lost or broken. Rodney Yee's other DVDs are also very good, including his one called *Yoga for Back Care* (Gaiam, 2003).

- *Anatomy for Yoga* by Paul Grilley.
  Topanga, CA: Pranamaya, 2014. ISBN 978-1585-65168-9; US$29.95.

  This best-selling four-hour comprehensive course is designed to help yoga students understand unique skeletal anatomy (every *body* is different!) and how the bones, joints, and muscles are affected by the physical poses in class. Re-released many times, I watched the 2004 edition as part of the anatomy portion of my yoga teacher training and it is still the best on the market. Grilley has a practical and intuitive understanding of body mechanics that is easy to comprehend for even a lay practitioner. Highly recommended for both circulating and professional collections.

- *Ashtanga Yoga: Primary Series—All Levels* by Mark Darby and Nicole Bordeleau.
  Montreal, QC: Productions Yoga Monde, 2003. ASIN: B0006I036C; Can$16.99.

  While there are many Ashtanga or "power yoga" DVDs on the market, this is the one I use myself and recommend over and over to my students and patrons. Not only does it offer short forms of the traditional ninety-minute primary series, but it features two simultaneous instructors (male and female) demonstrating the regular and modified-for-beginners versions of the poses. Plus the DVD is bilingual, giving you the choice of French or English.

- *Chakra Theory and Meditation* by Paul Grilley.
  Topanga, CA: Pranamaya, 2007. ISBN 1-934430-00-5; US$25.95.

  This five-and-a-half-hour DVD contains four hours of *Chakra* theory and ninety minutes of guided meditations broken into twelve practices, which serves as a great introduction to anyone wanting to learn more about the *Chakra* system and how it is affected by meditation and breath work. Not a necessary purchase but nice to have for the curious.

- *Good Morning Yoga: A Pose-by-Pose Wake Up Story* by Mariam Gates and Sarah Jane Hinder.
  Holland, OH: Dreamscape Media, 2017. ISBN 978-1520-06952-4; US$29.99.

  This twenty-minute video uses gentle movements combined with a sweetly illustrated narrative to get young children ready to face the day with more self-control and focus. It has a read-along feature, which is helpful for emerging readers and also serves as subtitles for the hearing impaired. An excellent addition to your juvenile DVD collection and also a great video to show during a morning yoga storytime program.

- *Goodnight Yoga: A Pose-by-Pose Bedtime Story* by Mariam Gates and Sarah Jane Hinder.
  Holland, OH: Dreamscape Media, 2017. ISBN 978-1520-06949-4; US$29.99.

  This seventeen-minute video is the perfect length to show during a yoga storytime or to recommend to parents who would like to introduce yoga to their young children. I gave it a test run with my five- and ten-year-old boys and it was (mostly) a success. The five-year-old was really into it and followed along with every pose; the ten-year-old was less enthused, as it is geared for a bit younger audience. It has a read-along feature to help emerging readers enhance their literacy, which also serves as subtitles for the hearing impaired. The tone is soothing and helps relax children (and parents) as they move through a series of breathing and movement exercises designed for beginners. While pricey for such a short video, it is worth adding to the juvenile DVD collection if you have room in your budget.

- *Shanti Generation: Yoga Skills for Youth Peacemakers* by Abby Wills.
  Woodland Hills, CA: Cinema Libre Studio, 2011. ASIN: B002FPX1CC; US$14.95.

  This DVD is geared toward youth ages ten to fifteen and contains five different thirty-minute practices, a library of poses, breathing and mindfulness exercises, and interviews with teen yogis. A great addition to your circulating collection or to purchase to use during teen programs. Share this one with high school teachers. Narration available in English, Spanish, and Japanese.

- *Yoga for Families: Connect with Your Kids* by Ingrid Von Burg, Tom Morley, and Gerardo Diego.
  Los Angeles: Bayview Films, 2009. ASIN B001M9PBK2; US$19.70.

  This popular thirty-minute yoga video is designed for kids ages four and up, though younger ones may find the transitions between each pose too quick. Engaging and lively, this DVD will circulate regularly.

ⓖ Designing Buildings and Spaces to Be More Conducive to Yoga and Meditation

Not all libraries, especially small ones, have the room for a dedicated yoga and meditation space. If you are lucky enough to be part of a renovation or new-building project, there are certainly resources to support the inclusion of these and other multipurpose programming spaces. I highly recommend checking out *3rd 4 All: How to Create a Relevant Public Space* by Aat Vos.[1]

Some public and academic libraries, as well as schools, offices, and even airports, are designating specific rooms for mindfulness, meditation, or yoga. These areas are for private or sometimes shared use (depending on the size of the space). They can either be silent, tech-free spaces, have TVs for playing yoga or meditation videos, or have soothing background music. The yoga room in the Burlington Airport in Vermont even has a shower across the hall, so you can work up a sweat while waiting for your flight.[2] The University of Kansas Libraries in Lawrence opened their third "reflection room" in August of 2018 at the request of the Muslim Student Association after students complained that there weren't enough appropriate places to pray on campus.[3] These rooms are basically retrofitted office spaces painted in soothing colors that contain no religious imagery, so they can be used by anyone for quiet contemplation.

When thinking about designing a meditation room in your own library, first see what sort of space you have available to carve out. Do you have an oversize closet that is large enough to be accessible for someone in a wheelchair? Or a small study room? It could be as simple as painting the walls calming colors, and putting a yoga mat and/or meditation cushion on the floor (and/or a chair for someone with limited mobility). If you have a larger space, you could have room for multiple mats or cushions, some blocks, straps, and other props, and perhaps even some books or digital devices for guided meditation. The iRelax space at the University of Toronto's Inforum Library combines all of these ideas to create "a secular, ethically and sustainably-sourced mindfulness resource area."[4] It offers yoga mats, cushions, wooden meditation benches, yoga blocks, and print resources available on a first come, first serve basis (on the honor system). They offer the following books in their mini-library (all good choices I highly recommend!):

- *Full Catastrophe Living: Using the Wisdom of Your Body and Mind to Face Stress, Pain, and Illness* by Jon Kabat-Zinn
- *Mindful Tech: How to Bring Balance to Our Digital Lives* by David M. Levy
- *Wherever You Go, There You Are: Mindfulness Meditation in Everyday Life* by Jon Kabat-Zinn
- *Yoga for Beginners: Simple Yoga Poses to Calm Your Mind and Strengthen Your Body* by Cory Martin
- *Yoga & Mindfulness Therapy Workbook for Clinicians and Clients* by C. Alexander Simpkins and Annellen M. Simpkins

At the information desk, students and faculty are able to check out noise-canceling headphones with iPods containing yoga videos or guided meditation instruction for an hour at a time.

The most important things to consider when making room in your library for yoga and/or meditation are:

- Is it relatively quiet, or can distractions be masked or minimized?
- If using for group classes, is there room for ten-plus people to move freely without hitting into walls, tables, support posts, bookshelves, chairs, and so forth?
- Is there storage space for mats and other props?
- Are the lights dimmable?
- Is it private, or can anyone walking around the library see in?
- Are the colors soothing and the space welcoming and inclusive?

If your potential or existing space doesn't meet these requirements, don't despair! As architect-cum-monk Phap Dung says in his introduction to Thich Nhat Hanh's essential little book *Making Space: Creating a Home Meditation Practice*, "Wherever people put attention and purposefulness into how things are designed, there's care and love in that space. . . . The intention of sacred space is to make room so we can return to ourselves and touch something deep within ourselves."[5] He goes on to remind us not to try to force our space into something it isn't, but to work with what we have to make it a place we have room to breathe in and be with ourselves and each other in the practice.

At my library our large multipurpose room is often used for yoga programs, and it is right next to the busy circulation desk, so even with the doors closed it is sometimes noisy. I remind students that this helps us practice with distractions. Here's some ideas to consider: Maybe you can play music (or a white noise machine) loud enough to drown out the background sounds? If you don't have enough space for a yoga program without people hitting into things, can you go outdoors? Is there a nearby green space or church/building with a vacant room you could use? Is there a way to rearrange the furniture to make it work? If you don't have room for dedicated mat and prop storage cabinets, can you repurpose an old book truck like I did? A cart on wheels also makes it much easier when the program needs to be moved to another section of the library! If your space has obnoxious fluorescent lights you can't dim, can you turn them off and add some sufficiently ambient lamps or battery-operated candles? If your space has windows, can they be covered so people can't see in? If it is in an open area of the library, can privacy screens be added? Or maybe you'll just have to accept a more open sort of atmosphere (or heck, just go right out on the front lawn). Can you offer programs off-site or online? Even after all these questions and ideas, if you still don't think you have the space, turn to chapter 5 to learn some sneaky ways you can offer yoga and meditation programs passively so you don't have to do any teaching at all! And then open up to chapter 11 to read about the many ways you can offer yoga and meditation programs off-site as outreach initiatives. Let's get creative!

⑨ Key Points

- There are several basic supplies most often used in yoga and meditation programs, like mats, cushions, and blocks, but costs can be kept low by finding creative solutions to funding and program delivery.
- Reputable sources for program supplies will often provide wholesale discounts to educators.
- Care should be used when purchasing supplies to make sure they are washable and that once acquired they are cleaned properly.
- Storage for program supplies must be considered before purchase and also whether the supplies need to be portable if they are being used for outreach services.
- There are many digital resources available for sharing with patrons and for training and program planning purposes.
- Creativity should be used when considering altering your existing spaces to accommodate yoga and meditation programs. There are examples available about what is working in other libraries to learn from.

⑨ Notes

1. Aat Vos, *3rd 4 All: How to Create a Relevant Public Space* (Rotterdam, Netherlands: nai010, 2017).
2. Ann Pizer, "Downdog on the Go in Airports with Yoga Rooms," VeryWellFit, June 14, 2018, https://www.verywellfit.com/airport-yoga-rooms-3566838.
3. Ronnie Wachter, "A Space Apart: College Libraries Contemplate Meditation Rooms," *American Libraries Magazine*, January 2, 2018, https://americanlibrariesmagazine.org/2018/01/02/library-meditation-rooms-space-apart/.
4. University of Toronto Libraries, "iRelax," Inforum Library, accessed November 9, 2018, https://inforum.library.utoronto.ca/spaces/iRelax.
5. Phap Dung, introduction to *Making Space: Creating a Home Meditation Practice*, by Thich Nhat Hanh (Berkeley, CA: Parallax, 2001), 9–10.

Passive Programs and Alternative Collections

IN THIS CHAPTER

▷ Defining passive programs and their purpose

▷ Understanding passive program delivery

▷ Exploring passive program models you can re-create in your own library

▷ Alternative collections to promote mindfulness

⟲ Defining Passive Programs and Their Purpose

PASSIVE PROGRAMS ARE ANY program initiatives that don't involve patrons participating at a set date or time but that can be done at their own leisure, either in the library (such as working on a puzzle) or as part of outreach services

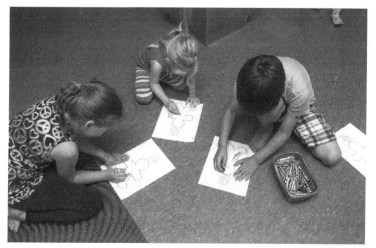

Figure 5.1. Mindful coloring pages make for an easy passive program. *Brendan Helmuth*

(such as taking home a coloring page from a library visit at a day care). They promote and encourage library resources and services, but incorporate minimal involvement or ongoing upkeep from staff, other than initial planning and implementation. Their purpose is to engage as many patrons as possible while working with limited staffing and operational time constraints.

⊚ Understanding Passive Program Delivery

Passive program delivery starts with an idea (or vague subject matter) and then finding a way to engage with a certain demographic. Such as wanting to do more meditation programs, and then figuring out whom to deliver them to. Or it could be the reverse, starting with an overlooked demographic and then thinking how to reach them using an enticing subject matter. For example, for early morning patrons who only stop in before work and can't stay long enough for a meditation program, you could offer them a bookmark at checkout with printed links to online resources and book/audiobook suggestions on the topic. The bulk of the work is done up front and behind the scenes. The program delivery is simply providing the materials and refreshing them as necessary, or removing them and replacing them with a new program. Different places in your library are good locations for passive programs, such as a designated space in your children's department, at your coffee shop (if you are lucky enough to have one), or in your study lounge. Passive programs can also be taken along during outreach initiatives and shared with attendees.

⊚ Program Models You Can Re-create in Your Own Library

Passive programs are really only limited by your imagination, budget, and the time you and your staff have to prepare them. At first you may think meditation or yoga would be impossible programs to offer in a passive format. How can people independently practice yoga or meditation, other than setting up permanent or semi-permanent spaces for them to do that, as we discussed in chapter 4? What if you don't have the room to create a yoga nook or meditation corner? Is it even safe for people to do yoga at the library on their own? Where do we even start? Here are five program ideas that are easily adaptable to a variety of settings and budgets. Have fun coming up with some of your own!

Wabi Sabi Wall

The Japanese term *Wabi Sabi* is something that is closely related to mindfulness and to Zen teachings. It is the willingness to leave things unfinished, or to accept yourself as unfinished; to appreciate the beauty of the world as it falls apart or deteriorates. Admiring a rotting log in the forest or leaving the hem of a skirt unfinished are very *Wabi Sabi* things to do.

Consider, then, the beauty that could be found by creating a *Wabi Sabi* wall at your library. It could be a wall of words and drawings that are unfinished for people to work on and leave their mark, such as a large piece of butcher paper spread across a surface and access to pencils and erasers. Or a large metal surface with a magnetic poetry kit for people to make impromptu haikus. The heading could say: "Learn to embrace the imperfect!" or "Where I want to be is where I am." Leave it at that and see what people come up with.

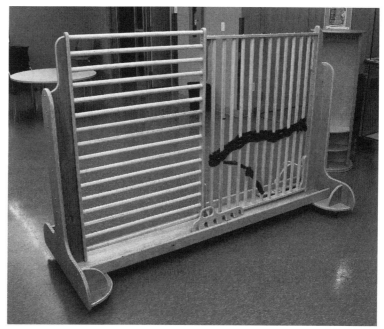

Figure 5.2. A weaving wall on wheels for portable program play.
Brendan Helmuth

At our library we have something called a weaving wall. It is a wooden structure that looks like an oversize, simplistic loom and there are nearby buckets filled with scrap fabric and ribbon. We keep it in our children's department, but it is on rolling casters so we can take it outside to use it for programming with natural fibers (such as leaves, grasses, and flowers) in the summer. Children (and their parents!) come along and weave the materials through the loom, creating impromptu art pieces that are promptly destroyed by the next curious soul who comes along and repurposes the fabric for their own design. It is very *Wabi Sabi*—never finished, never perfect—always in the process of changing into something new, but nevertheless beautiful.

To complement your *Wabi Sabi* wall, consider making a display of related materials. Here's some ideas to get you started:

A Little Book of Japanese Contentments: Ikigai, Forest Bathing, Wabi-Sabi, and More by Erin Niimi Longhurst and Ryo Takemasa

Perfect Imperfect: The Beauty of Accident Age and Patina by Karen McCartney

Simply Imperfect: Revisiting the Wabi-Sabi House by Robyn Griggs Lawrence

Wabi Sabi: The Art of Everyday Life by Diane Durston

Wabi-Sabi for Artists, Designers, Poets & Philosophers by Leonard Koren

Wabi Sabi: Finding Beauty in Imperfection by Oliver Luke Delorie

Wabi-Sabi: Further Thoughts by Leonard Koren

Wabi Sabi: The Japanese Art of Impermanence by Andrew Juniper

(*continued*)

Wabi Sabi Love: The Ancient Art of Finding Perfect Love in Imperfect Relationships by Arielle Ford

Wabi-Sabi Sewing: 20 Sewing Patterns for Perfectly Imperfect Projects by Karen Lewis

Wabi Sabi: Timeless Wisdom for a Stress-Free Life by Agneta Nyholm Winqvist

Wabi-Sabi Welcome: Learning to Embrace the Imperfect and Entertain with Thoughtfulness and Ease by Julie Pointer Adams

Wabi-Sabi Wisdom: Inspiration for an Authentic Life by Andrea M. Jacques

Wabi Sabi for Writers: Find Inspiration, Respect Imperfection, Create Peerless Beauty by Richard R. Powell

Yoga and Mindfulness Card Decks

Yoga and mindfulness card decks are something I have been using in programs for years. They make great prompts for activity planning; kids love to follow along with the cards during free play or use them to show other kids their mad yoga skills. The yoga cards especially are a great visual alternative to traditional text-based books for encouraging physical literacy in reluctant readers. Plus, they are fun!

If we think outside the box (pun intended!), card decks can also be used as adaptable resources for passive programming and/or alternative collections. You can buy a number of decks, catalog them, and allow them to circulate, as you would any other title. They make for beautiful and interactive displays (and gifts and bookmarks!). But you can also just buy some decks and put them out in common areas of your library. There are decks available for children, teens, and adults. Scatter the boxes of cards around the library, perhaps with a little label or standing sign saying what they are for, and allow people to feel they have permission to use them. The next thing you know you'll find a dad doing an impromptu Down Dog with his daughter, or two teens giggling over pictures of plucky pumpkins, or a stressed-out student taking a break with a meditation exercise. Will they get ripped, broken, stolen, and lost? Yup. But with an average price of $16 a box, they are affordable enough to replace for most budgets. As an alternative, you could always get crafty and design and laminate some of your own!

Here are some reviews of decks I have personally used and recommend, with suggestions of how to use them in both independent and structured programming:

The ABCs of Yoga for Kids: Learning Cards by Teresa A. Power and Kathleen Rietz. Pacific Palisades, CA: Stafford House, 2010. ISBN 978-0982258736; Card deck; US$19.95/Can$21.95.

This popular children's book is also available in a flash-card format that is great for self-directed learning. Each card has a pose corresponding with the letter of the alphabet ("S" for "Slide," for example) that kids and caregivers can try out on their own, with written instructions on the back. Pictorial instructions would be more helpful, but these are still worth purchasing to put out for a passive program. If using during storytime, get every student to pick a card and go back to their mat to try it out (putting aside the more difficult ones if you are teaching the toddler crowd). They can then switch with a friend. Another fun option is to have someone pick a card from the deck and "be the teacher." They get to come up to the front of the room and teach the rest of the class how to do the pose on their card and everyone can try it out together (warning: this may not appeal to introverts!). I've done it as an icebreaker activity with adults/staff, and everyone gets a good giggle while feeling awkward.

Be Mindful Card Deck for Teens by Gina M. Biegel.
Eau Claire, WI: PESI Publishing, 2016. ISBN 978-1-55957-058-9; Card deck; US$16.99/Can$22.75.

This card deck is great to put out in the young adult department in a public library, to use during a teen mindfulness program, or to have in a high school library (especially during exam time!) or even in the classroom (lend them out to teachers). It can even be added to an alternative collection of card decks if your library has one. Like any item left out for patrons to use, the cards may deteriorate over time, or get stolen, but at $16.99, the cost is minimal if your teens are getting some stress-relieving benefit out of them. The fifty cards come in three different types: sensory based, relationship based, and ones for getting "unstuck" or switching gears. The design of the cards is very hip, with lots of artsy, geometric shapes and soothing colors, which will appeal to image-conscious teens. Here is an example of one of the exercises: "What do you taste in your mouth right now? Even if you think nothing, what does nothing taste like?" There are also "wild cards" that are blank for students to create their own ideas. You could photocopy these and make this into a program: students can come up with their own favorite mindfulness exercise to keep in their wallet or purse.

How Am I Feeling? Conversation Cards by Saxton Freymann and eeBoo Corporation
New York: eeBoo, 2018. ISBN 978-1-68227-152-0; Card Deck, US$11.99/Can$14.99.

These cards are worth buying just for Freymann's adorable award-winning artwork. Featuring fruits and vegetables carved to demonstrate different emotional expressions, these flash cards can get kids talking about their feelings and helping to develop empathy for other people's experiences. As a mindfulness tool, these fifty cards can spark an internal dialogue about the acceptance of our vast range of emotions and serve as a jumping-off point to talk to others about them. Each facial expression has a prompt on the back of the card to encourage conversation or self-reflection. Also a great literacy tool, the cards can be used in programs to promote storytelling or writing exercises. For example, on the back of a card with a kiwi yawning the prompt is, "Is this kiwi ready to go to work or ready to go to sleep? How do you know when you are tired?" This can generate a discussion about self-care routines, recognizing when others are tired and don't want to play, telling stories about sleep and rest.

(*continued*)

I Heard Your Feelings Conversation Cards by Saxton Freymann and eeBoo Corporation
New York: eeBoo, 2017. ISBN 978-1-68227-055-4; Card Deck, US$11.99/Can$14.99.

More analytical and advanced than the *How Am I Feeling?* deck reviewed above, these fifty cards feature situational drawings of cartoon animals on one side and interpretive storytelling prompts on the other side. Designed to foster empathy and improve social skills, these cards can help children (and adults) learn to be more mindful when interacting with others. Complex social dynamics, societal expectations, and navigating our own tricky emotions while interacting with others can cause stress, and these cards can give patrons helpful practice using the tools of mindfulness. For example, one card features a rabbit holding up a birthday present with a look of consternation on its face while the giver—a pig—looks on in disappointment. The prompts include: "Does Rabbit like the gift from Pig? How does Pig feel? What should Rabbit do? Why does Pig care about Rabbit's reaction?" These cards make a great addition to preschool storytime themes involving feelings or values (such as sharing or telling the truth) and can also be put out in common areas for passive interaction. The scenes can also be acted out for dramatic play or used as prompts for storytelling, writing, or other literacy programs.

Mindful Games Activity Cards: 55 Fun Ways to Share Mindfulness with Kids and Teens by Susan Kaiser Greenland and Annaka Harris.
Boulder, CO: Shambhala, 2017. ISBN 978-1-61180-409-6; Card deck; US$19.95/Can$25.95.

These cards are full of program ideas to be used in a public or school library as part of existing programs or combined for stand-alone events. They are also useful for passive programming in your children's or teen department, or anywhere youth congregate. Each card has a consistent, accessible format listing the following: the duration of the game (most are three to fifteen minutes), the age level (young children, older children, teens, all ages), instructions for leading the game (including helpful talking points), tips, and variations or modifications. They are well worth their reasonable price. I would buy a copy to put out for patrons *and* a copy to keep to use for programs and program planning.

Mindful Kids: 50 Mindfulness Activities for Kindness, Focus and Calm by Whitney Stewart and Mina Braun.
Cambridge, MA: Barefoot Books, 2017. ISBN 978-1-78285-327-5; Card deck; US$14.99/Can$19.99.

The box claims these cards can be used by anyone aged 4–104, and it's true! Highly enjoyable, the funky, detailed illustrations alone are enough to keep anyone flipping through them even if they don't do the exercises—which they should, because they are really fun and engaging. The cards come with a trifold insert explaining what mindfulness is and why it is useful and explains how the cards are divided into five categories: Start Your Day (to stay grounded and confident from the beginning), Find Calm (to ride the waves of tricky emotions), Focus (to build sensory awareness), Open Your Heart (to accept life with kindness), and Rest and Relax (to ease your monkey mind). There's an important note about modifications and how anyone, with any body type or limitation, can practice mindfulness. It includes helpful tips for what to do if you feel uncomfortable, physically or emotionally, during the exercises. The cards echo this inclusive sentiment by including illustrations of children from all different ethnicities, and includes a child in a wheelchair. These cards would be fine to use for passive programming, but they also spark lots of ideas for activities! An example of one of the exercises is called "Open Ears" and is an activity designed for two or more people and requires a bell, chime, or something that makes a "ding!" sound. The children are asked to sit quietly in a circle and choose a leader. The others close their eyes and take three mindful breaths, and then the leader rings the bell. Everyone listens to the sound of the bell as the ring slowly disappears; then they raise their hand when they feel like the sound is totally gone. Then everyone listens for the other sounds in the environment. The leader rings the bell again, and everyone opens their eyes and shares what they heard with the group. This exercise builds mindful listening and turn-taking skills, and creates links between the auditory system and the focusing parts of our brain (prefrontal cortex).

Yoga Planet: 50 Fun Activities for a Greener World by Tara Guber, Leah Kalish, and Sophie Fatus.
Bath, UK: Barefoot Books, 2008. ISBN 978-1-84686-181-9; 50 cards; US$14.99.

I took my children's yoga teacher training with Leah Kalish, who is one of the authors of this card deck, which I then purchased after my training to use in my classes. There are fifty cards (mostly physical poses) with decent explanations and good illustrations to help children (and adults) play with them on their own. But be warned, there are also some fairly useless cards with suggestions for activities like riding your bike instead of taking the car (not like many kids have a choice in this matter) or using "rainbow power" to send good thoughts to a friend. These cards will largely be ignored by your patrons (but they make good bookmarks!). The games and partner poses, on the other hand, like "Doorway" or "Over & Under," are extremely useful. I have yet to figure out why this card deck is for a "greener world" other than the "Earth, Air, Fire, Water" theme that will go largely unnoticed by all but the most discerning of yogis, and the occasional trite environmentally conscious–themed card. That said, all in all, this is a good deck to have on hand and has been well loved by my own children and many students over the years, so it is not without merit.

Walking Labyrinth

If you ever visit a meditation retreat center, at some point you will more than likely be asked to do some walking meditation. That walking meditation will often involve walking slowly and mindfully in circles. If sitting still for long periods of time in silence wasn't enough to numb your monkey mind into obedience (or insanity), I can assure you walking round and round and round as slowly as humanly possible will do it (if only temporarily!). There is something incredibly calming about walking; many famous writers and intellectuals have been known for their long, rambling excursions. In fact, it is a common stim (stimulation activity that calms the nervous system when experiencing sensory overload)

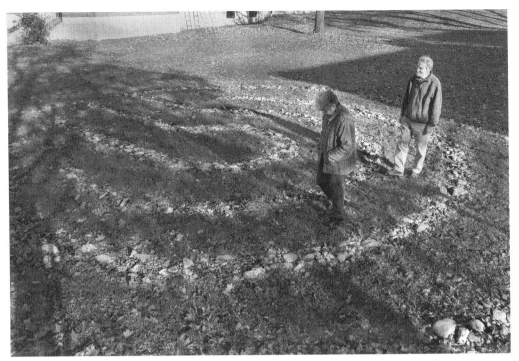

Figure 5.3. Elderly couple walks in stone and grass labyrinth. *Brendan Helmuth*

among those with sensory processing disorders (such as those on the autism spectrum) as well as the general public (think of the common image of a frantic father-to-be pacing back in forth in front of the delivery room door). In other words, walking mindfully seems to be something that calms humans down.

I often include walking elements into meditation classes (and which are included in many program models in this book), but sometimes it is nice to allow patrons to move in contemplation at their own pace and in their own time. One way to do this is by working with your municipality to create a walking labyrinth. Here in Woodstock, NB, we are lucky enough to have a stone and grass labyrinth and a peace pole installed in a green space on the same block as the library. We can recommend it to patrons or use it as part of our programs. We don't have a large enough lawn of our own, since we are in a downtown location and real estate is at a premium, but a more rural library or those with bigger garden spaces could create a walking path of their own. If your town has self-directed walking tours, you could ask to have the library and your labyrinth included. If you are at a school or university library, talk to your administration to see if there is available space on campus.

If outdoors is not an option due to space restrictions or weather (and here in New Brunswick the winter lasts six to seven months, so I have empathy), you can purchase a canvas version for using indoors. Portable, easy to clean, and relatively lightweight, a walking labyrinth made from washable poly duck canvas can be purchased online from retailers such as Labyrinth Company.[1] While not durable enough to be left out year-round, they can be brought out during special events, holidays, or exam time, and even taken on the road to use when doing outreach programs. The only problem is their price tag. Starting around US$1,000, they are definitely an investment. Some libraries have acquired them through wellness grants or other funding. It is worth looking into what is available because they are sure to be popular with patrons of all ages. Make sure to put up a sign explaining their significance so people feel they have permission to use the space and know what to do with it.

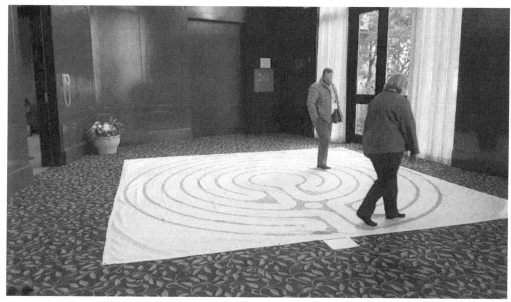

Figure 5.4. Indoor walking labyrinth. *Madeleine Charney*

Interactive Stations

Depending on your type of library and budget, you can use your creativity to come up with all sorts of interactive stations that encourage independent moments of mindfulness. In an academic, medical, or law library you could preload an iPad with meditation or yoga apps and have it locked to a desk in a quiet study area for patron use. You could also consider installing a soothing water fountain and plants near individual seating that encourages quiet contemplation. A mini Japanese-style Zen meditation garden, complete with miniature rake and stones, can be purchased and left out for stressed students and faculty to play with. In public or school libraries, where kids are more likely to make a mess, you can substitute the regular sand for the commercial sensory play sand that is easier to clean up. Instead of a water fountain you could have bottles filled with water and glitter or small lightweight toys in water for students to shake and swirl. Watching the glitter fall is very soothing.

Coloring stations are also a very popular form of relaxation in both public and academic libraries. Set out some pencil crayons, markers, and some mandala coloring sheets. There are many adult coloring books on the market for you to choose from, or free images you can print off the internet. At our library we even have a weekly adult coloring group that meets up every Friday afternoon to color for a few hours together. We just put out the supplies, but they often bring their own and then all go out for coffee together afterward. Sometimes we play soothing music, and sometimes they bring snacks. It's the easiest program ever and they love it. Everyone is welcome, and it takes absolutely no time to prep other than setting out the materials.

Mindful Movie Club/Yoga Movie Club

Do you have a large DVD collection? Why not put out a display of movies to do with mindfulness and meditation and/or yoga? As part of the display, include a bulletin board with blank recipe cards and a few pens. Encourage patrons to check out the items, and when they return the materials they can write mini-reviews of the titles on recipe cards, which you can pin to a bulletin board above the display.

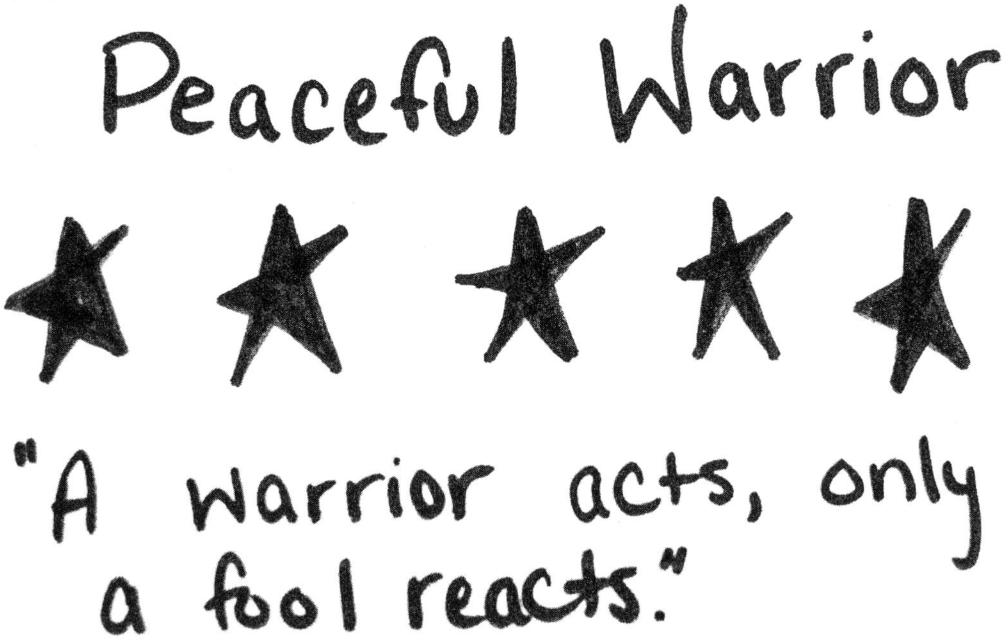

Peaceful Warrior

★ ★ ★ ★ ★

"A warrior acts, only a fool reacts."

Figure 5.5. Use index cards for patrons to rate the films. *Ebony Scott*

Mindfulness Movies

Here is a list of mindfulness-based films (fiction and non-fiction) to get you started on your display:

Being in the World (2010)

Dalai Lama Awakening (2014)

Dalai Lama Renaissance (2007)

The Dhamma Brothers (2008)

The Examined Life (2008)

I Heart Huckabees (2004)

Inner Worlds, Outer Worlds (2012)

Into Great Silence (2005)

The Mindfulness Movie (2013)

On Meditation (2016)

One, The Movie (2005)

Peaceful Warrior (2006)

Waking Life (2001)

Walk with Me (2017)

What the Bleep Do We Know? (2004)

Yoga Movies

Here are some instructional or entertainment-based yoga DVDs—bonus points for the increase in circulation statistics!

Ashtanga Yoga: The First Series (2008)

Breath of the Gods (2012)

Easy Yoga for Arthritis with Peggy Cappy (2010)

Eat Pray Love (2010)

Element Prenatal & Postnatal Yoga (2009)

Enlighten Up! (2008)

Kundalini Yoga: Healthy Body Fearless Spirit (2011)

Kung Fu Yoga (2017)

Rodney Yee's Yoga for Beginners (2009)

Shiva Rae Core Yoga (2012)

Yin Yoga: The Foundations for a Quiet Practice (2005)

Yoga for Families: Connect with Your Kids (2009)

Yoga Hosers (2016)

Yoga Is (2012)

Yogawoman (2011)

Alternative Collections

While a detailed explanation of how to process and establish non-traditional circulation collections in your library service is beyond the scope of this book, there are many fine resources available on the topic.[2] As a supplement to existing mindfulness programs, or to encourage independent practice and reach a wider audience, I suggest adding some of the following items to your circulating collection of non-book objects—dependent, of course, on your institution's policies on (and tolerance of) alternative collections:

- Meditation cushions
- Meditation kits: includes cushion and CD or preloaded device with guided meditation
- Meditation or yoga card decks
- Passes to local yoga studios
- Yoga kits: includes a mat, block, strap, and instructional DVD
- Yoga mats

⊚ Key Points

- Passive (independent) programs are a great way to reach a wider patron audience with minimum input from staff.
- Passive program models are only limited by our own creativity and can be modified for various budgetary situations, audiences, and institutional settings.
- Passive programs can supplement or complement existing programs or act as stand-alones.
- Passive programs can help promote circulating collections.
- Alternative format collections (libraries of "things") are another way to promote yoga and meditation in your community without creating and delivering formal programs.

⊚ Notes

1. Labyrinth Company, "Poly Canvas Mats," Labyrinth Company, accessed November 10, 2018, https://www.labyrinthcompany.com/collections/poly-canvas-mats.

2. American Library Association (ALA), "Non-traditional Circulating Materials," Public Library Association, accessed November 12, 2018, http://www.ala.org/pla/resources/tools/circulation-technical-services/nontraditional-circulating-materials.

CHAPTER 6

Policies and Procedures for Avoiding and Handling Problems

IN THIS CHAPTER

▷ Identifying potential legal issues and creating policies and procedures to protect your staff and patrons

▷ How to handle other potential problems or special issues

▷ A checklist of required forms and policies for all programs

---

◎ When Things Go Wrong and How to Prevent It

IN ORDER TO TEACH yoga and meditation programs in libraries, we need to first think through any potential mishaps or misunderstandings that may arise so that we can both prevent them and also mindfully and skillfully deal with them should they occur. This chapter will attempt to identify any of these issues so that you can go about creating strong boundaries (i.e., written and enforced policies and procedures) around these topics of concern.

◎ Liability Insurance

It is very important for anyone teaching yoga (or any movement-based program) in a library to have liability insurance, and important also for the patrons to be covered under the building's insurance, should someone get injured during a class. You can check with your current insurance policy to see if staff and volunteers are covered. Personal liability insurance is usually less than $200 per year, and proof of it should be a requirement for all outside teachers coming to facilitate programs in your branch. Often staff and patrons may be covered under your existing blanket policy, but outside teachers will likely not be. Yoga Alliance offers a discount to US members through Alliant Insurance, and in Canada a popular source for insurance is through Lackner McLennan, which you can purchase by visiting www.yogainsurance.ca.[1]

Criminal Record Checks

Criminal record checks, specifically ones for the vulnerable sector (disabled, elderly, youth), are to confirm that potential employees or volunteers have never been convicted of a criminal offense. They are something most libraries in Canada require and are becoming more common in the US. Drug testing may also be required. Keep in mind that these letters are not guarantees that your potential teacher has never committed a crime or is a good person. Conducting a thorough interview, checking teaching certifications (such as graduating from a Yoga Alliance–certified yoga teacher training program), and calling applicable references is highly recommended.

Hold Harmless/Liability Waivers

It is absolutely essential to have every patron (or their parent/guardian) sign a liability waiver (also known as a hold harmless agreement) to absolve the library and its staff of responsibility should the patron suffer an injury during a movement-based program. Patrons should also be advised not to begin any sort of exercise program without first visiting their doctor to get the OK. Keep in mind this won't guarantee absolution of potential guilt should an incident undergo litigation, but it will work in your favor. If you have a recurring program at your library (say, a yoga class every Wednesday evening), patrons only need to sign the form once, at their first class, but make sure it stipulates on the form the dates of the program and that it is ongoing. Regardless if it is the same faces every week, it's always a good idea to check in with students at the beginning of class to see if they've acquired any injuries or recent illnesses that you may need to offer modifications for. This also applies to positive body changes, such as pregnancy, as you will also need to modify the poses to accommodate their evolving state. You can find samples of liability waivers used for library programs at http://letsmovelibraries.org/resources/.[2]

Photo/Video Release Forms

Whenever we want to grab a few photos or a video of patrons involved in our programming, it is essential to have them (or their parent/guardian) sign a photo release waiver.[3] If you have patrons whose first language isn't English, make sure to explain clearly what they are signing and what is going to happen to the photos. Be mindful that not everyone wants to have their photo taken (especially while wearing stretchy pants and contorting their body into compromising positions). While library staff do need to make an effort to document programs and work harder on promoting services, we also need to be careful to not undermine the whole premise of a yoga and meditation class, which is to give people a safe space to unwind and feel less exposed to judgment. Your patrons don't want to show up and feel like they need to perform—or be on display for the judgmental eyes of your Instagram followers—they need a community space to be themselves with their imperfect bodies and imperfect monkey minds.

The "Religion Issue"

One controversy that may come up from patrons, staff, and administration is whether yoga and meditation are a "religion" (or related to a specific religion) and therefore shouldn't be offered in a government-run institution like a public or school library, or in a faith-based university or school. As discussed in previous chapters, the movement-based *Hatha* yoga we are practicing in libraries is only one branch of yoga. The physical poses were designed—an estimated two thousand years ago—to help yogis be able to sit for long periods of meditation. Meditation, as we also learned in previous chapters, is a contemplative practice that helps train the mind to cultivate more awareness (also called mindfulness), which promotes mental and physical well-being. This meditation, like prayer, was and is used by different religions such as Buddhism, Hinduism, Jainism, Islam, and so forth, but that does not mean that meditation, and the physical yoga *Asanas* cannot be practiced and presented in a secular fashion.

At any of the libraries or schools I've taught yoga and meditation, this has rarely been an issue, especially once I explain the above information in an understanding way to the concerned patron or parent. Sometimes Facebook posts for our library will get negative comments about our yoga programs being "the devil's work," but I either delete those comments or urge those commenters to visit the library to check out our wide selection of books on the topic to educate themselves about the history of yoga and meditation. I've been very fortunate that it's never gone any further than that. It's good to remember, as Dan Harris points out in *10% Happier: How I Tamed the Voice in My Head, Reduced Stress without Losing My Edge, and Found Self-Help That Actually Works—A True Story*, some people may attempt to argue that yoga and meditation will erode the practitioner's primary faith, but if packaged, delivered, and practiced from a secular standpoint, as should be done in libraries or any publicly funded community center, then yoga and meditation simply become a tool for mental hygiene.[4] Meditating does for the mind what flossing does for the teeth. In fact, as Harris articulates, perhaps quieting the voices in our head can actually help us feel closer to whichever God or deity we believe in.

Touch and Consent

Not everyone likes to be touched. Not by strangers, and sometimes not even by people they love and trust. You don't know people's personal history, you don't know what kind of trauma they are carrying in their body, and you don't know how they will react to your well-intentioned—perhaps unknowingly unwanted—help. Don't assume because you would like an adjustment during a yoga class that your student would also. Other people desperately crave touch and will be disappointed if they feel like you aren't helping them to get their alignment "just right" in a pose. You may be inclined to not bother (why take the risk?), but many students claim this as the favorite part of the practice—this chance to be touched in a calming, non-sexual way—and to *be seen and accepted* on their mats, just as they are.

There is much controversy in yoga circles over whether or not hands-on adjustments can be therapeutic or are potentially re-traumatizing.[5] Friendly, nurturing touch releases feel-good hormones in the body, such as oxytocin, that promote bonding and trust between two people and lower our heart rates. But when we've experienced touch as something invasive and threatening in the past, our neurobiology may override our system's normal responses and instead code touch—any touch—as unwanted, perhaps even downright dangerous. This leads to a vicious cycle of social isolation, mind-body disconnection, and mistrust. The unconditional positive regard formed between teacher and student in a yoga or meditation class may be the first step in bringing a traumatized person to a place of healing, but we want the pace to be set by the student and not the teacher.

First off, you need to decide, as a teacher, how comfortable you feel touching your patrons. You must be honest with yourself: Will you touch everyone equally? Will you pay special attention to the people in class you know better, or who are your friends? Will you be tempted to linger longer on that patron you've always had a little crush on? Will you avoid touching the smelly student with the unwashed hair? Check your own bias before you even begin teaching. If you can't give physical adjustments and modifications fairly, don't give them at all. Also, do you have enough training to give proper adjustments? An excellent resource is Mark Stephens's *Yoga Adjustments: Philosophy, Principles, and Techniques*.[6] Practice at home with friends and family until you feel comfortable and confident enough to give adjustments to strangers.

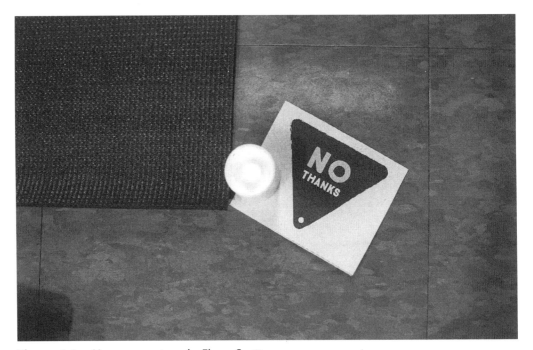

Figure 6.1. Yoga consent cards. *Ebony Scott*

Keep in mind that patrons may be too shy or uncomfortable to say in front of everyone that they don't want an adjustment. When I give adjustments during *Savasana* (also known as Corpse Pose, a complete resting position), I always wait until everyone's lying down with their eyes closed before I say, "If you don't want me to touch your feet or neck, please put your hands on your belly." That way no one can tell who is opting out. Another great option is to use consent cards. These paper cards are handed out at the beginning of class, and people can put them at the front of the mat indicating whether they would like adjustments. This makes it more private and gives the student a feeling of autonomy.

If you aren't the one leading the class, make sure to have this conversation with any hired or volunteer facilitators so everyone is on the same page.

Another option I like to offer is for students to safely touch themselves. When leading a loving-kindness meditation, for example, I will ask them to bring their right hand to their heart, or when breathing deeply in *Savasana* I will ask students to place a hand on their belly "without judgment." This closes the circle of trust and helps remind students that they are always there to love and support themselves, so they are never truly alone.

When leading mindfulness programs that may touch on sensitive subjects, such as grief or other pain points, I ask the students at the beginning of the session to give me a "thumbs-up" if they have to leave the room for any reason. Just so I know they are OK. If they don't give me the symbol, I'm going to assume they are upset and need help, and I will follow them out of the room (or send my assistant) to check on them. This also builds trust.

Teaching What You Know

This comes back to the importance of training, which we discussed thoroughly in chapter 3, but I'd like to touch on it again for a moment. If you don't feel comfortable teaching something, and know deep down you aren't qualified, don't do it. Your authenticity is your number one asset. This also applies to asking staff to teach programs they may not feel qualified to teach, which is why open conversation between management and employees is so vital to the health of your workplace.

I feel comfortable leading programs that may involve trauma recovery, physical and cognitive disabilities, and mental health issues because I've been trained in suicide first aid and prevention, non-violent conflict resolution, intervention for those with sensory processing disorders and behavioral problems, and other mental health protocols. But, for example, I have absolutely no business leading a workshop on transcendental meditation, because I've never done it before. That's when I would call a trained facilitator to come lead the program. Your teaching will change as you continue your education and personal practice, and you will learn to adapt it accordingly, but teach for who you are today, not who you hope to be tomorrow. Trust it will come.

When Accidents Happen

Make sure you have incident report forms handy to keep a record of any injury that may occur during a yoga class. Even if you just jot down what happened to the student, and have any available witnesses sign it, it could prove very useful should that student later return claiming that they've suffered lasting damage due to an injury they received during a library program. If something major happens, such as someone having a heart attack during class, make sure after immediately dealing with the emergency you also offer debriefing to the other people who witnessed the event, such as students, staff, and volunteers.

Pregnant Students

What happens when a pregnant student shows up for your regular (non-pregnancy-themed) yoga class? First you should check with the student (privately) to make sure they've had the OK from their doctor to exercise, and if they have any complications. After that it is a good rule of thumb that anyone in their first trimester should avoid yoga, or only do the gentlest forms, because the fetus is still implanting and the risk of miscarriage is highest.[7] All pregnant students should breathe through their mouth and avoid most *Pranayama* (breathing exercises), twists, and lying on their backs or bellies. If you don't have any training or experience teaching pregnant students, get some, because pregnant people will show up and it would be unconscionable to ask them to leave.

Students with Exceptionalities

Like with pregnancy, students with physical or cognitive disabilities should be welcomed to class like everyone else. Modifications to suit their particular needs should be provided easily and without embarrassment to the student. If you don't feel you have the proper training to provide this, make sure you add it to your continuing education plan, and in the meantime recruit a facilitator who does have the training to make modifications.

Dress Codes

What people wear to a yoga class may differ from what they wear in the rest of your facility, and your dress policy, should you have one, must reflect that. For example, it might be perfectly reasonable to expect everyone to wear shoes in your library, but you don't want people wearing shoes on your yoga mats. You might not even want them to wear socks. But some people's religion, culture, or personal sense of propriety may prevent them from exposing their feet in public. When it comes to the topic of how to dress for yoga programs, we need to be culturally sensitive. Every region of the world has its own culturally sanctioned dress for "public" and "private" (which can be interpreted as "casual"), and sometimes "exercise clothes" can cross between those two territories. Opinions about this even vary tremendously within cultures, even within families. If you work in a culturally diverse library, you may have people who show up for a movement-based program wearing everything from short-shorts and belly shirts, to hijabs, saris, sweatpants, or full Amish garb. I usually recommend that students wear comfortable clothing that allows me—the teacher—to see the major joints of the body (knees, hips, elbows, shoulders, ankles, wrists) so that I can make verbal or physical adjustments, as necessary. This can be done by either wearing form-fitting clothing that hugs the joint (e.g., mainstream yoga pants) or shorter, looser clothing (e.g., shorts that end just above the knee). That said, I allow any clothing in a yoga class so long as the practitioner is meeting the public decency laws, which may be very different where you live. For example, in my province, nipples are required to be covered for males and females in a library building, so no one may take off their shirt during class, even if they get sweaty. In the province of Ontario, women are permitted to be topless in the streets, the same as men, but inside government facilities or parks they are required to cover their nipples. It's a fine line. If you are doing yoga outdoors in Ontario and it isn't in a park, can students go topless? I suggest you familiarize yourself with your laws and facility's policies. If you are teaching in a school library setting, more than likely there is a dress code already in effect. If your library doesn't have a dress code policy, do you want one? If so, who will enforce it?

The reality is that yoga is exercise, often done in somewhat binding clothing, and wardrobe malfunctions happen. As a yoga teacher going on her second decade in the business, I've seen my share of exposed thongs, see-through leggings, testicles peeping out of too-short shorts, bulging breasts, and more. People also pass gas in class, sometimes by mistake and are incredibly embarrassed, or sometimes exuberantly with good humor. Teaching yoga is not for the prudish or easily offended. That said, it is *your* job to create good boundaries in the class and set a professional example. If someone's behavior or clothing (or lack thereof) is making everyone uncomfortable, by all means speak to them about it (privately) after class. Also think about what you are wearing at the front of the room, as you set the tone. I suggest your clothing should cover as much skin as is comfortable, and refrain from having large logos or abrasive messages, since you are still at work and are representing your institution. You want people coming for the yoga, not to see the librarian-yogi in a state of undress.

Resisting the Urge to Enlighten

My personal practice, at work and at home, is to try to give people as much room to grow as possible. And mostly that means keeping my mouth shut. People won't listen to 99 percent of your "helpful" advice anyway. Even though they will undoubtedly ask. People sometimes put yoga and meditation instructors on the same pedestal as medical doctors or psychologists, and will ask you all sorts of questions about how to fix their problems, which you are totally unqualified to answer. Even if you are also a medical doctor. Because when you are practicing as a yoga teacher, you don't need to be answering questions about how to treat bronchitis. As service-oriented people, we like to help, but as Anne Lamott gently reminds us, help is often the sunny side of control.[8] Let it go. Whenever you get the urge to help people reach some level of consciousness you think you can get them to (because, of course, you have it all together, right?), read my favorite advice from Zen teacher Shunryu Suzuki:

> Even though you try to put people under control, it is impossible. You cannot do it. . . . To give your sheep or cow a large spacious meadow is the way to control him. So it is with people: first let them do what they want, and watch them. This is the best policy. To ignore them is not good. That is the worst policy. The second worst is trying to control them. The best one is to watch them, just to watch them, without trying to control them.[9]

People Being People

Above all else, as librarians, we are very adept at handling people being . . . well . . . people. So I already know you can do this, because you do it all day long. People are going to do stupid things that don't make any sense. They are going to occasionally put themselves and others at risk, or at least annoy the heck out of everyone in a twenty-foot radius. They are going to shock you and gross you out, in all their human glory. Things don't get any less hairy because everyone's trying to be all Zen'd out in yoga or meditation bliss. If anything, people will show up for these classes in their most raw versions of themselves and we need to be prepared for it. Have tissues—there will be crying. Have policies and procedures about age requirements for classes and prepare yourself mentally for how you are going to handle enforcing them. Because you *will* have that mother who doesn't speak English show up with two toddlers to an adult yoga class, and when you try to explain as best you can with your hands that the children aren't welcome, she won't understand and will calmly watch her children run around the legs of everyone trying to do a precarious balancing pose, not because she's a jerk, but because she just doesn't understand the protocol and you can't explain it. Things will get lost in translation. This, of course, will also happen with people who *do* understand English, or any language you speak, and *don't care at all*, and this is 100 percent more irritating, because they are being jerks. Godspeed.

You will see lots of underwear poking out of stretchy pants, or worse, pants that are so see-through you wish there was underwear underneath them. People will fart and burp during class. They will laugh obnoxiously and talk among themselves. They will get up and leave with no explanation or walk in halfway through the class and demand a mat or ask you where the bathroom is. They will cough their way through thirty minutes of meditation and resist your polite offers of water or throat lozenges. They may complain through the entire class—loudly. They may try to give you tips or flowers you can't accept. They may ask you out. They may say things like, "Wow, a sexy librarian *and* a yoga teacher!" Or, "I can't believe *you* teach meditation, you're always so stressed out." But they will also be funny and grateful and curious and supportive and the best part of your day. People will keep on peopling, and you are going to keep doing what you do best: serving them the best you can, with the tools you have.

CHECKLIST OF ESSENTIAL PAPERWORK

○ Liability/hold harmless forms (for patrons/volunteers/teachers)
○ Photo/video release forms (for patrons/volunteers/teachers)
○ Incident/injury report forms (for patrons/volunteers/teachers)
○ Yoga consent cards (for patrons)
○ Liability insurance (for volunteers/teachers)
○ Criminal record checks (for volunteers/teachers)

⊚ Key Points

- It is essential to have written policies and procedures in place *before* offering yoga and meditation programs at your library and training your staff on how best to enforce them.
- Liability insurance is essential for anyone teaching a movement-based program in your facility or off-site on your behalf.
- All teachers and volunteers must have clean, up-to-date criminal record checks for working with the vulnerable sector before teaching.
- Hold harmless forms (also known as liability waivers) need to be signed before anyone can participate in a movement-based program.
- Photo/video release forms need to be signed before photos or videos can be taken of any patron.
- Yoga and meditation are not religions, though they are used by different religions. All yoga and meditation programs presented in this book are secular in nature and can be done by anyone, regardless of their religious background.
- All touch provided by teachers in class should be consented to first by the student, and students have the right to change their mind about wanting to be touched at any point during the program.

- Teachers should only teach things for which they have proper training and feel comfortable delivering. This includes ensuring others only teach things for which they are qualified.
- Incident report forms should be completed and reviewed whenever someone experiences an accident or injury during class.
- Pregnant students should be welcome in class, and poses need to be modified to suit their special needs.
- Students with physical or cognitive disabilities should also be welcome in class and modifications provided to suit their needs.
- It's a good idea to establish some sort of dress code for yoga classes and to make patrons aware that it may differ from the dress code elsewhere in the building.
- Yoga and meditation teachers will often be solicited for advice that they are not qualified to deliver and should resist offering opinions on medical issues, such as injuries, or otherwise.
- It is important to remember when teaching yoga and meditation programs in libraries that they involve people and people can be unpredictable. Establishing strong policies and procedures while also being adaptable and having a sense of humor is the most practical approach for mindfully serving your community.

Notes

1. Yoga Alliance, "Alliant Insurance," Yoga Alliance, accessed November 10, 2018, https://www.yogaalliance.org/AlliantInsurance; Lackner McLennan Insurance LTD, "Yoga Liability Insurance," Yoga Liability Insurance, accessed November 15, 2018, https://www.yogainsurance.ca/.

2. Let's Move in Libraries, "Safety First," Let's Move in Libraries Resources, accessed November 15, 2018, http://letsmovelibraries.org/resources/.

3. You can find a sample photo release form from my library service here: Government of New Brunswick, "Appendix A: Standard Photo Release Form," *The New Brunswick Public Library Service Policy 1017*, January 2018, https://www2.gnb.ca/content/dam/gnb/Departments/nbpl-sbpnb/pdf/politiques-policies/1017_UseOfPhotos_Appendix.pdf.

4. Dan Harris, *10% Happier: How I Tamed the Voice in My Head, Reduced Stress without Losing My Edge, and Found Self-Help That Actually Works—A True Story* (New York: Dey Street Books, 2014).

5. Suzanne E. Jones, "Mindful Touch: A Guide to Hands-On Support in Trauma-Sensitive Yoga," Yoga Service Council, 2018.

6. Mark Stephens, *Yoga Adjustments: Philosophy, Principles, and Techniques* (Berkeley, CA: North Atlantic Books, 2014).

7. Arielle Nash-Degagne, "Prenatal Yoga: The Essential Guidelines for Practice," Love Yoga Anatomy, accessed November 16, 2018, https://loveyogaanatomy.com/prenatal-yoga-the-essential-guidelines-for-practice/.

8. Anne Lamott talks about this concept in many places, but a nice introduction comes from reading the transcript of her hilarious and enlightening TED talk (or watch the video): "12 Truths I Learned from Life and Writing," tinyTED, accessed November 16, 2018, https://en.tiny.ted.com/talks/anne_lamott_12_truths_i_learned_from_life_and_writing.

9. Shunryu Suzuki, *Zen Mind, Beginner's Mind: Informal Talks on Zen Meditation and Practice* (Boulder, CO: Shambhala, 2011).

Yoga and Meditation for the Early Years

Yoga and Meditation for Babies, Toddlers, and Preschoolers

YOGA AND MEDITATION PROGRAMS geared toward babies, toddlers, and pre-schoolers are as much for their caregivers as for the children themselves. I mean, have you ever watched toddlers stick their bottom in the air—full on Down Dog–style? They are already like little yogis. And there is nothing more Zen-like than well-fed babies staring off in space as they drift off to sleep. Children at this age are all about living in the moment. As Joseph Chilton Pearce says in *Magical Child*, "There are no big or little events to the two-year-old, all is breathless excitement, awe and wonder."[1] So when we design yoga and meditation programs for this age group, our participants' natural curiosity can lead the way. Especially when designing programs for babies, we are often focusing on the needs of their caregivers, while also giving their children opportunities for gross and fine motor development, as well as introducing them to early literacy concepts. We are teaching the caregivers a literacy framework they can replicate at home (choose books with high contrast illustrations; read often; use songs, rhymes, and fingerplays; etc.). I recently attended a workshop on the maternal mental health benefit of preschool storytimes while presenting at the Next Library Conference in Berlin and

▲ 49

wasn't surprised to learn that mothers who attended specially designed library programs had significant improvements in their perceived well-being, even if they were ostensibly attending for their children's edification.[2] The combination of community, acceptance, creativity, structure, accomplishment, and fun is enough to boost the moods of both parent and child. For those of us who have been working in libraries for a while, it is no secret that libraries are good for the health and well-being of our patrons (of all ages), with improved literacy just being one of many benefits.[3]

Program Models

Below are three program models. One is a yoga class designed for mothers and their babies. Another is a play-based story hour that uses hands-on art activities and story-telling to introduce the concept of mindfulness to children aged three to five. And the last program combines traditional fairy tales with their twisted versions to explore the concepts of yoga and mindfulness with preschoolers. While these last two programs aren't specifically designed for toddlers (ages one to three), they can both be modified for that age group. The discussions following the stories will be slightly less sophisticated (or in the case of late talkers, non-existent), and you may want to shorten the program to only twenty to thirty minutes. Other suggestions are offered in the "Advice" section of each program model. The most important thing to remember with teaching yoga and meditation to the littlest students is to have fun and not take it too seriously. We're just planting the seeds that will grow into tomorrow's knowledge!

Program Model: Mom & Baby Yoga

Before you start with the whole "This is not gender inclusive!" or "What about grand-parents/nannies/caregivers/aunts, etc.?!" outrage, let me explain that this program is *not*

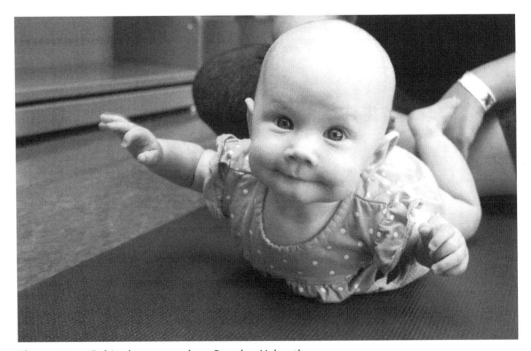

Figure 7.1. Babies love yoga class. *Brendan Helmuth*

baby yoga, it is a program designed for the post-partum reintegration of a mother's pelvic floor. That doesn't mean the babies won't love it. But the babies are more like props. It gives moms a chance to get out of the house and do something social and self-caring that doesn't require hiring a babysitter. Does that mean that an adoptive mother can't bring her little one? No. Does that mean a dad (or same-sex non-birthing partner) isn't welcome? Of course not. It's the library—everyone is welcome! Just make sure to explain clearly in the marketing material that this program is going to be focusing on rebuilding the inner core muscles that get damaged naturally during pregnancy and childbirth and *is not* a yoga class to help babies be more flexible. Have you watched babies suck on their toes with ease or Zen out staring at dust motes? They've got this yoga thing down already. It's the moms who need this class. Though, as an added benefit, as the mother's heart rate decreases, and the room settles into that magical *Savasana* calm, the babies will naturally bliss out too. Don't believe me? Try it for yourself!

Advance Planning

Step 1. Either find a teacher who is familiar with post-partum yoga, or if you are teaching the class yourself, familiarize yourself with the sequence (see pages 54–55) and run through it a few times.

Step 2. Pick a day and time for the event. We surveyed local moms and found that morning sometime between ten and eleven (we open at ten) was best because many of their babies napped in the afternoon and/or the moms had to be home to greet older children after school and get dinner ready. We settled on 10:30–11:00 on Tuesdays. You don't want the program to last longer than thirty minutes, because that's about the length of time the babies will be willing to cooperate and you want the experience to enhance their mothers' well-being, not detract from it. We do book the room from 10:30 to 11:30, so that the moms can stay afterward and socialize and not feel like they need to rush out because the room needs to be set up for another program. And that way, if all the babies are cooperating, we can sneak in a little more yoga or a longer *Savasana*.

Step 3. Decide whether this will be a one-off program or an ongoing weekly or monthly event. We tried it once, just to see what the response would be, and it was so overwhelmingly positive that we decided to make it a weekly program. You also need to decide if it is going to be drop-in or registration only. Decide how many pairs you will accept. Remember some mothers may bring toddlers or other children along. Is this OK with you? Is there room for everyone?

Step 4. Book the room you will be using. Space may play a factor in how many people can attend. We have two different spaces we've offered the program. One is in the big open play space in our children's department. It isn't the quietest space, but it works because we're close to nursing chairs, the washroom, and the board books so that we can remind parents to take some home afterward. Also, if parents bring older children along there is space for them to run around and play. The drawback is it is out in the open and some moms may feel self-conscious doing yoga or breastfeeding in full view of other library patrons. The other space we use is an activity room with tinted windows and doors we can close. It has an attached bathroom, which is nice, and is more private than the other space. The downside is there are no comfortable nursing chairs and it can get booked up quickly for other programs. Figure out what works best for you and don't feel shy about soliciting feedback from your audience.

Step 5. Make sure you have all the required materials (see list below).

Step 6. Advertise your event. Make a print poster. Make a Facebook event. Put it on your website and event calendar. Tweet about it. Share a photo of an adorable baby on Instagram with details about the program. Visit local day cares and schools to drop off a poster for families to see. Visit your local mom and baby playgroup to talk about it. Share the event with local family doctors, churches, and anyone else who may come into frequent contact with families with babies. And make sure to tell every mom and baby pair who comes up to the reference or circulation desk. Word will spread fast. Our first post on Facebook received more than seventeen hundred views in two days—not bad in a town of fewer than six thousand people!

Step 7. Do the paperwork. Make a sign-up sheet if you require registration. Prepare liability waivers. Prepare photo release waivers if you plan on taking photos/videos of the event.

Materials Required

- Yoga mats
- Foam or cork yoga blocks (thick books will do in a pinch)
- Beanbags
- A teddy bear or doll
- A singing bowl or bell
- A board book to read at the end (*Goodnight Moon* by Margaret Wise Brown and Clement Hurd or *I Am Yoga* by Susan Verde and Peter H. Reynolds or *Bedtime for Chickies* by Janee Trasler are some good choices)
- Liability waivers
- Photo releases and camera (if using)
- Clipboard and pens (for signing waivers)
- Baby wipes
- Copies of infographic (see pages 54–55) for everyone to take home
- Evaluation forms for final session

Budget Details

$0–$500. The budget for this program varies greatly depending on if you have to buy the mats and blocks and other supplies. Most public libraries have beanbags, a camera, a teddy bear/doll, and clipboard on hand. If you can't get yoga blocks, just use thick trade paperbacks (hardcovers are too heavy). If you can't afford mats, you can always do this program right on the large children's play carpet (assuming you have one) because none of the poses are done in standing, so there's no risk of slipping. Grants to purchase equipment or hire instructors are often available through wellness agencies, sports associations, or post-natal health programs. If you need a teacher, see if you can recruit a volunteer through your local yoga studio.

Day of Event

Step 1. Prepare the room by setting out the mats and props. Get your waivers and clipboard ready.

Step 2. Greet your moms and show them where the washroom is located as well as the nursing chair (if there is one available) and invite them to have a seat on one of the mats and get comfortable. Welcome everyone to share their names, their babies' names, how old their babies are, and one special memory they have from the last week. Say something like, "Wow, getting out of the house is so hard when you have a little one, I'm so impressed you made it!" This helps improve maternal mental health and gives them an opportunity to feel proud of their accomplishments as new moms.

Step 3. Once everyone has arrived, explain that the class is going to focus on the pelvic floor, which are the deep inner core muscles that hold up the internal organs. These muscles get stretched out to accommodate the growing baby and subsequent delivery. Make sure all the moms are at least six weeks post-partum (eight weeks if they've had a C-section or other major complications). If not, invite them to watch the class so they'll know what to do. Show them how to check to see if they have diastasis recti (see sidebar for more info) and advise them to follow up with their doctor if they do. Tell them the intention for the class is for them to be *gentle, patient, and persistent* with themselves. They may have anxiety about getting back into shape after having a baby; reassure them it takes time and is totally possible if done in a healthy way that minimizes the chance of injury.

HOW TO TEST FOR DIASTASIS RECTI

Have your students lie on their backs, with their knees bent and feet on the floor. Tell them to place one hand palm down over their bellies, with their fingers pointing toward their toes. Ask them to press their fingers gently into their belly button while slowly lifting their head, drawing chin to chest, in a mini-crunch. This causes the rectus abdominis to contract.

If there is a gap of at least two finger widths between the muscles as they contract, there may be a diastasis. A gap as wide as four or five fingers is considered severe. The separation may be wider in different places, so they should repeat this procedure above and below the belly button. If they find a gap they should consult with their general practitioner or a physiotherapist.

Step 4. Invite the moms to lie down on their mats, feet flat on the floor, and put their babies on their bellies. If their baby is asleep in the carrier, give them a teddy bear or doll or beanbag to use. If they have twins, have them take turns with each baby. Reassure them that the babies may not always cooperate and that is fine. Encourage them to nurse, take breaks, or leave if they need to. Ask them to let you know if they feel any sharp, shooting pain, and to stop immediately.

Step 5. Go through the sequence in the infographic (pages 54–55), encouraging them to take nice big belly breaths, slow and steady, and not to worry what anyone else is doing on their mat. If their baby spits up or cries, just keep going, or stop to offer them a baby wipe.

Step 6. At the end of the sequence have everyone sit on their mats, babies in their laps, and read your chosen story, encouraging them to take a few board books home. Let them know that books with simple language and high visual contrast (like black and white) are great for babies. Use a soft, lightly lilting voice to help lull the babies (and moms). After *Savasana*, have everyone close their eyes and take a deep breath, and ring the bell. Alert them that they may be slightly sore tomorrow from all the pelvic floor work and that it might feel a little funny when they pee because they worked the same muscles

Mom & Baby Yoga

with Jenn Carson

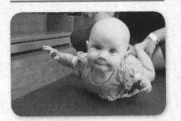

This gentle sequence is designed to help new mothers work on postpartum reintegration of their pelvic floor muscles. You should wait at least 6 weeks (8 weeks if you had a cesarean or any major complications) and get approval from your doctor during a postnatal check-up before participating.

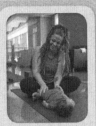

1. Introduction
Today we're going to be gentle, patient, and persistent with ourselves. You may have some anxiety about getting back into shape after having a baby, but know that it takes time and we're going to approach it in a gentle way that minimizes your chance of injury. Take a comfortable seat on your mat and give your baby some nice gentle rubs (if they are awake).

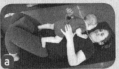

2. Pelvic Floor Pose (a) Come into lying on your back with your baby (or a bean bag) on your belly. Your feet are planted on the floor with your knees pointing toward the ceiling. Place a block between your thighs and squeeze to activate the pelvic floor muscles. Inhale and feel your baby lift toward the ceiling. Exhale, pull your belly button down toward the ground. Repeat 5 times. (b) Tuck your chin and curl your upper body into a crunch position. Hold your baby with your hands so they don't slide off. Inhale and use your tummy muscles to raise your baby toward the ceiling. Exhale and pull the belly down, lowering your baby. Squeeze the block with your thighs. Repeat 5 times.

3. Leg Crunch (a) Raise your knees to a 90° angle and sit your baby up against your knees, if that's ok for their neck. Keep your head and shoulders on the floor. Inhale and lift belly. Exhale and squeeze the block, lowering your belly. Repeat 5 times. (b) With knees still raised to a 90° angle, squeeze the block and lift your upper body off the floor. Look toward your baby. Inhale and lift your belly. Exhale and lower your belly. Repeat 5 times.

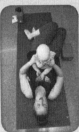

4. Knee Twist Remove the block from between your thighs and lower your feet to the floor. Drop both knees to one side, keeping your baby on your belly and your shoulders/head planted. Take 5 breaths. Repeat on the other side.

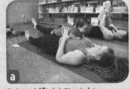

5. Leg Lift (a) Straighten your legs and hold your baby on your belly. Lift one leg a few inches off the floor and hold the position for 5 breaths. Lower the leg and repeat on the other side. (b) Repeat (a), but this time raise your head and shoulders off the floor while you lift your foot. Engage your tummy muscles and hold for 5 breaths for each leg lift. If this is too hard on your neck, repeat (a).

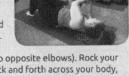

6. Shoulder Twist While lying on your back, plant your feet on the floor with knees pointed toward the ceiling. Hold your baby in your arms (or clasp opposite elbows). Rock your arms and baby back and forth across your body, keeping your torso planted on the ground. If it feels good for your neck, you can turn your head and watch your baby as you rock them back and forth. Repeat 5 times on each side.

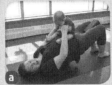

7. Modified Bridge Pose (a) Place the block between your thighs with your knees bent and feet planted on the floor. Your baby can sit on your belly. Hold on tight, they are going for a ride! Lift your bottom off the floor, squeezing the block with your thighs. Take 5 belly breaths and then lower down slowly.
(b) Repeat (a), but this time squeeze the block and lift one leg, straightening it as much as you can. Keep your hips in the air for 3 breaths and then lower down. Repeat on the other side.

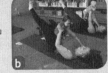

www.jenncarson.com • www.yogainthelibrary.com • www.physicalliteracyinthelibrary.com

Figure 7.2.

Mom & Baby Yoga

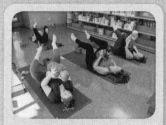

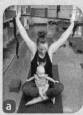

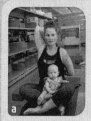

8. Leg Rotations Lying on your back, lift your legs in the air while holding your baby over your torso. Rotate your lower legs, making large circles, toward the outside walls of the room, alternating legs so you don't bang your ankles together. After one minute, go the other direction, with legs rotating toward the center.

9. Shoulder Strap Stretch (a) Sit in easy pose with your baby in your lap. Holding the strap in your hands at a comfortable distance for your shoulders, reach your arms overhead. Lower your arms in front of your torso. Repeat 5 times. (b) Still sitting in easy pose and holding the strap, raise your arms over your head. Tilt your arms to one side, leaning with your torso. Lift your arms back overhead and lower on the other side. Repeat 5 times on each side.

10. Cow Face Pose (a) Sitting in easy pose with your baby in your lap, hold the strap in your right hand. Reach your right arm above your head and let the strap dangle down your back. Reach up with your left hand from behind and grab the strap. (b) Walk your fingers toward each other until you feel a good stretch. Hold for 5 breaths. Repeat on the other side.

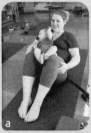

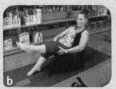

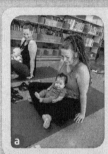

12. Uplifting Pose (a) Cross your ankles and place your baby in your lap. Place your hands on the floor beside your hips. Lift your seat off the floor. (b) Option to place blocks under your hands to make it easier. Hold for 10 breaths.

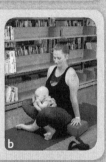

11. Boat Pose (a) Sit with your knees bent and your feet flat on the floor, holding your baby in your lap (if they will cooperate!). Grasp the back of your knees. (b) Inhale and lift one leg to the same height as your chin. Exhale and lower. Repeat on the other side. Then try with both feet lifted. Repeat the whole sequence 3 times.

13. Child's Pose (a) Kneel on the floor with your knees spread wide. Place your baby on the floor facing you (or optional tummy time!) with your arms outstretched. Take 5 deep breaths.

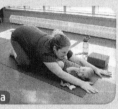

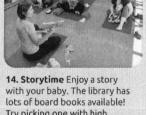

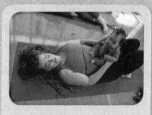

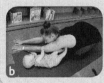

(b) Walk your hands to the left to stretch out your intercostal muscles. Take 5 breaths. Walk your hands to the right, take 5 more breaths. Come back to center.

14. Storytime Enjoy a story with your baby. The library has lots of board books available! Try picking one with high contrast (like black and white) illustrations. *Goodnight Moon* by Margaret Wise Brown or *The Very Hungry Caterpillar* by Eric Carle are classics. Reading to your baby now will help develop a lifelong love of literature.

15. *Savasana* Now it's time for *Savasana* and a snuggle. Lie on your back with your baby on your belly or next to you (option to keep knees bent and feet flat on the floor). Drop your breath into the lower lobes of your lungs and breathe deeply. Your baby will feel your calmness. Close your eyes. Stay for as long as you'd like.

Program design by Jenn Carson • Photography by Drew Gilbert • Layout by Brendan Helmuth

Figure 7.3.

that control the flow of urine. Invite them to return to the next session and remind them of the day and time (unless this is a one-off).

Step 7. Clean up. Offer them a handout of the infographic to take home to continue their practice on their own time. If this is the final class in a series, hand out a short two- or three-question evaluation to be completed, but don't take it personally if they rush out and don't complete it; they have a mini-person who needs their immediate attention or appointments they can't miss. Hang around in case anyone has any questions or concerns they wanted to ask you about privately. Invite the moms to stay and socialize as long as they'd like to (if this is an option in your space)—the program is just as much about giving moms a social wellness opportunity as a physical one.

Advice

- Remember, you are a yoga teacher–librarian, not a medical doctor (unless you are *also* a doctor—double fist bump). This means you cannot, nor should not, diagnosis possible conditions. But you can let them know they exist, like diastasis recti. People will ask you to anyway. The proper response is, "I'm sorry, I'm not a doctor. But I can help you find a book on the subject after." No sense wasting those precious opportunities to boost circulation stats.
- Don't forget the baby wipes. There *will* be spit-up on the mats. And possibly poop, so have a disinfectant handy. If you couldn't handle puke or poop, you wouldn't be working in a public library anyway.
- It would be great to have a display of post-partum yoga books and DVDs nearby to refer to and/or a handout with a list of links to digital resources.
- A word of caution: don't take talking during the class to mean the moms aren't interested. Remember, for a lot of new parents, this might be their only opportunity that day to have another adult to chat with, and they relish the chance for connection. Same goes if they are late or leave early. Congratulate them for making it out of the house and show empathy for the difficulties of having little ones. Take nothing personally.
- Some moms with newborns will show up even though they are not six to eight weeks post-partum. You can recommend they don't participate until they get the OK from their doctor and have waited the required amount of time, but they may try to do the class anyway. When this happens I just teach the class and let them do their own thing. They've signed a liability waiver. They've been told the risks. Your administration may have a different view on the matter, so it is always best to check.
- The babies may startle and even cry when you ring the bell. This means their startle response is working! They will get used to it. If it bothers you, or the mothers, you can do something gentler, like humming "Om" softly or using a rain stick.
- For more resources and suggestions about running baby-centered yoga programs, please visit www.yogainthelibrary.com or read my blog post on the subject at Programming Librarian: http://www.programminglibrarian.org/blog/yoga-baby-steps.

Program Model: Little Minders

A great way to introduce mindfulness concepts to preschoolers is by using storytelling (frankly, this works well with big kids and adults too!). Little Minders is a program designed for parents/caregivers and their children aged three to five. It's a thirty-minute program that involves a carefully chosen picture book or oral story, a group discussion, a focus object, and a very short meditation (two to three minutes) with optional sharing afterward and a chance for creative expression. There are a number of excellent picture books that can be used for this program; this one is designed to be used with *Open in Case of Emergency* by Richard Fairgray and Jim Kraft. You can find other recommended mindfulness-based picture books listed at the end of this chapter or at my website: www. physicalliteracyinthelibrary.com under "Book Reviews." If you'd like to make this a recurring program, use the same format with a different book and do a craft or activity associated with the book you've chosen. There are activity suggestions included in the reviews.

Advance Planning

Step 1. Read the book and familiarize yourself with the story, since it will be central to your mindfulness activity. *Open in Case of Emergency* tells the story of two neighbors, Zachary J. Warthog and Cyrus P. Rhinoceros, who both receive mysterious boxes on their doorsteps one day. The small wooden boxes have a hand crank on the side and are labeled with bright red block letters that spell, "Open in Case of Emergency." Zachary Warthog proceeds to open his box that very same morning while he is making breakfast and runs out of sugar. He turns the crank, and out pops a packet of sugar, ending his crisis. He goes on to use the box over and over to remedy various predicaments until one day he loses it. Cyrus Rhinoceros takes the opposite approach: when catastrophe strikes, like a snowstorm or a tornado, he reasons that whatever he is dealing with is probably manageable after all, and decides not to use the box. When his neighbor frantically explains he's lost his emergency box, Cyrus calmly offers him his box. Zachary opens it to find his own missing emergency box inside. The story ends with the friends walking into the house arm in arm.

One of the most important lessons mindfulness has to teach us is to let other people be themselves. This is called *unconditional positive regard*. We don't force our opinions and advice on other people, or judge them for not making the same decisions we do, or having the same reactions we have. In the story Cyrus is allowed to relate to the emergency box in his hesitant, thoughtful, safeguarding way and Zachary is allowed to relate to his box in a more interactive, attached, trivial way. One neighbor clearly has a very different interpretation of the word "emergency" than the other. Most importantly, there is no judgment made on behalf of the authors over which method is better; the protagonists are simply allowed to have their stories. Each character shows a great deal of reverence for his box, but one approach is to use it constantly, the way a small child might carry around a much-loved toy, and the other refuses to use it at all, the way another child may put a special item up on a high shelf to keep it safe. After you read the story, be prepared to discuss these concepts with the children in your group. Sample questions are listed under "Day of Event" below.

Step 2. Decide what day and time you are going to offer the program. Since it is geared toward three- to five-year-olds, a weekday or weekend morning would be good, since most children that age still nap in the afternoon.

Step 3. Reserve the room you are going to use for your program. Do you have sit-up-ons (cushions) available for the children to use and chairs in the back of the room for the parents, unless they want to join you on the floor? Will it be a drop-in program or require registration? Do you need to make a sign-up sheet?

Step 4. Gather the necessary supplies (see "Materials Required" section below for a handy checklist) and decide whether you want to make the origami boxes or the drawing. These boxes are where they are going to draw or put their imaginary emergency items.

Step 5. Prepare the "emergency" focus box. This is a box you will use for your mini-meditation. Decorate it to look as fancy as you'd like. You could try to replicate the one in the story, or take a completely different approach (glitter! feathers! gemstones! faux leather!).

Step 6. Advertise your program through Facebook, Twitter, print posters and calendars, and the usual channels. Consider inviting local day care groups to join, if you have the resources. Don't forget to invite your local homeschool families.

Materials Required

- *Open in Case of Emergency* by Richard Fairgray and Jim Kraft[4]
- Small box (preferably labeled "Open in Case of Emergency")
- Singing bowl or bell
- Blank paper and pencils or crayons
- Scissors (if making origami boxes, unless you have square origami paper)
- Cushions for sitting (if using)
- Photo release forms and camera (if using)

Budget Details

$0–$20. The biggest expense for this program will be purchasing a copy of the book (US$16.99), but hopefully your library system already has a copy, or you can order one through interlibrary loan (ILL). A small box is easy to find in the recycling bin, and you probably already have the other craft supplies on hand. If you don't have a singing bowl or bell, use a free app on your phone.

Day of Event

Step 1. Welcome everyone to the program and explain the format: story, discussion, short mindfulness session, and a craft (this timeline is as much for the parents as it is for the children). Have them sit in crisscross applesauce (Easy Pose) on the floor (or cushions). Parents/caregivers can join in, or sit on the chairs available.

Step 2. Read the story and ask the kids some questions as each topic comes up (be prepared for some adorable answers and expect this to take much longer than you would expect). Everyone should get a turn to share, if they want to, but don't let any one child dominate the conversation. You can also wait to ask all the questions at the end. Here are some ideas to get the discussion going; feel free to add your own or adapt as you go:

1. What do you think is an emergency? Name a time you felt you were in an emergency. What did that look like or feel like to you?
2. Do you have a special object at home? How do you treat that special object?
3. How do you act or feel when other people are having an emergency?
4. How do you treat other people's special objects? If you knew your brother/sister/parent had an item that meant a lot to them but you didn't think it was all that great, how would you act around them and their object?

Step 3. After your discussion, have everyone sit in a circle and put a special-looking box in the middle of the circle. Ask the participants to sit quietly and stare at the box and imagine what could be inside. Invite the parents/caregivers to join you on the floor. Ask everyone to think about their answer while taking deep breaths (model deep breathing for them using exaggerated breaths). Have them sit up nice and tall with their hands on their knees. Tell them to keep breathing but not to say their answer out loud, that there will be time to share at the end of the meditation. Breathe a few more breaths until you can tell from their squirming they can't take it anymore and then ring the singing bowl or bell to bring them out of the meditation. Don't be surprised if they erupt into silliness.

Step 4. Have them raise their hands to take turns telling what would be inside their own emergency box. Have them guess what is inside yours.

Step 5. Use the remaining program time to offer the children paper and pencils or crayons to draw their own emergency boxes and the object(s) inside. This gives an opportunity for less verbally expressive students to share their internal processes. If you are feeling especially ambitious, you can have them fold their paper into an origami box and put their imaginary emergency objects inside.[5]

Advice

- If children have a hard time sitting up nice and tall, ask them to slump over and try to take a breath like that. Ask them if they notice it is harder to breathe when bent over. This may encourage them to sit up straight.
- If the children are having a hard time focusing on their breath while looking at the box, ask them to notice the cool air as it comes in through their nose and the warm air as they breathe it out. Many will make huge exaggerated breaths; let them do that for a minute and then for contrast ask them to stop and to try breathing "normally" and to focus on that.

⊚ Program Model: Yoga Fairy Tales Storytime

In this fun program designed for children aged three to five, you will read an original fairy tale then read a "twisted version" and do some yoga poses afterward. Maybe even ones

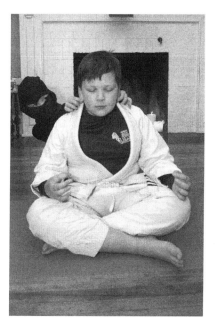

Figure 7.4. Ninjas and martial artists meditate too.
Ebony Scott

with lots of twists! If you can manage to sneak in some discussion questions to promote mindfulness among your young charges—double bonus points! This flexible (pun intended!) program format allows you to add it into an existing preschool storytime, modify it for an older or younger audience, or use as outreach when visiting schools, day cares, parks, or other places children want to hear a story and move their bodies! An element of dramatic play can be added by providing some costume props at the end for free play or making some masks or animal ears as a craft activity. Have fun!

Advance Planning

Step 1. Read the books and familiarize yourself with the stories. Here's a list of three program model suggestions to get you started.

YOGA FAIRY TALES BOOK PAIRINGS AND POSES

Program 1: *Little Red Riding Hood* (traditional) and *Ninja Red Riding Hood* by Corey Rosen Schwartz and Dan Santat.[6]

Decide which version of *Little Red Riding Hood* you'd like to tell based on the age of your audience. A Latin manuscript from 1022 contains the original story of a red-cloaked girl who is taken by a wolf but is unable to be eaten because of her red cloak. Charles Perrault first published (in French) a version for adults where the girl unknowingly eats her own grandmother at the costumed wolf's invitation but later escapes through her own cunning. In 1812, the Brothers Grimm version has the little girl being devoured, but later saved by the Woodsman. More modern versions have Red running out the door for help once she realizes Granny is actually a wolf and the Woodcutter comes to her aid, either scaring the wolf until he spits out Granny whole or cuts her out of his belly. You decide which version you'd like to tell to your storytime group. Some parents may bristle at a gorier version, even if the kids don't seem to mind.

Ninja Red Riding Hood is a twist of the classic fairy tale, one where our wolf just can't seem to catch any prey, so he takes some martial arts training to see if he can't upgrade his hunting skills. Confident with his new kicking and punching skills, the wolf journeys into the forest and comes across a little girl going to visit her grandma. Just like in the traditional tale, the wolf sneaks ahead but this time discovers her grandma isn't home, so he dresses up like her (lipstick and all!) and crawls into her bed. Red is having none of it, as is to be expected, and our wolf soon discovers that Red has been to ninja school too! They tussle and appear to be evenly matched, when suddenly Red's grandma arrives (in her gi, from tai chi!) and this gives Red the confidence boost she needs to put the wolf in his place. Thoroughly defeated, the wolf concedes he is no match for the lady warriors, and promises to become a vegetarian. The three make friends, and the wolf heads off to a yoga retreat where he gives up red meat, stops fighting, and finds peace at last.

Yoga pose suggestions: Down Dog, Warrior sequence, Goddess Pose, Lumberjack Pose (see "Yoga for Heartache" infographic in chapter 11 on page 147, for example).

Activity suggestions: Make wolf masks or ears, make ninja masks, play hide-and-seek with the person who is "it" wearing a wolf mask or (for the twisted version) a red cape.

Program 2: *The Boy Who Cried Wolf* (traditional) and *The Wolf Who Cried Boy* by Bob Hartman and Tim Raglin.[7]

The story of the shepherd boy who cries false alarms until no one believes him and his sheep are eventually eaten by a real wolf is one of Aesop's famous fables.[8] *The Wolf Who Cried Boy* is a delightfully twisted version your students (and parents!) will enjoy about a little wolf who doesn't want to eat his mother's cooking so he sends his parents chasing after imaginary boys until one night a whole Boy Scout troop comes by and they don't believe him.

Yoga pose suggestions: Down Dog, Cat/Cow, Lion Pose, Triangle, and Revolved Triangle Pose.

Activity suggestions: Decorate sheep shapes with cotton balls, play tag with the "wolf" wearing ears and chasing the sheep, create "Mama Wolf meals" with plastic play food or playdough.

Program 3: Humpty Dumpty (traditional) and *After the Fall: How Humpty Dumpty Got Back Up Again* by Dan Santat.[9]

Oh, poor Humpty Dumpty! We all know the classic nursery rhyme of how he fell off the wall, into many pieces . . . but what happened after? Well, it turns out all the king's men *were* able to put him back together again . . . sort of . . . with bandages and glue. But H.D. is so traumatized from the experience that his life has never been the same. In *After the Fall* we learn he can't, for example, seem to climb back up his favorite wall to watch the birds, which used to be his most enjoyable pastime. But one day, determined to overcome his fear of heights, H.D. tackles the ladder up the wall, and discovers once he reaches the top that he is no longer afraid. He knows that accidents can happen, but he has also learned that he can survive them. An important lesson to us all, and a great opportunity to discuss how to overcome challenges with your students. Try giving them a really challenging balancing pose (or even just standing on the blocks with one foot) and practice falling and getting back up. The magic twist at the end of the story is that Humpty hatches on top of the wall and turns into a magnificent bird who flies away, no longer afraid of heights. He hopes he'll now be remembered as the "egg that got back up" and not the one who was famous for falling.

Yoga pose suggestions: Crane, Peacock, Pigeon Pose, King Pigeon, Firefly Pose, Tree Pose.

Activity suggestions: Egg decorating, wall building with yoga blocks or plastic/wooden toy blocks, decorate a phoenix with colorful feathers.

Step 2. Recruit a yoga teacher if you aren't planning on teaching the class yourself and go over the chosen books and program plan.

Step 3. Decide on a time and date and if the program is going to be a recurring event. This is a good program for those trepidatious staff members who may wish to try teaching a yoga class but are also nervous. Just pick one or two poses to incorporate into an existing storytime format. Mornings are good for this age group and their caregivers.

Step 4. Reserve the room.

Step 5. Decide if you'd like to add a craft or dramatic play element and if so, prepare the craft and/or gather the necessary costumes and supplies.

Step 6. Gather all other materials required, as listed below.

Step 7. Prepare liability waivers, photo release forms, and a registration sheet (if using).

Step 8. Advertise the event. Make a poster and add to print and online calendars. Share with day care groups and homeschool families. Share on social media accounts.

Materials Required

- Depending on which program model you've chosen, the necessary books
- Craft supplies, if using
- Dress-up supplies, if using
- Yoga mats and blocks, if using (not necessary, but helpful if available)
- Singing bowl or bell
- All required paperwork and camera (if using)

Budget Details

$0–$100+. Assuming you already have access to most of these books, this could be a fairly cost-free program. If you need to buy the books and hire a yoga teacher, it's going to run close to $100 or more. If you want to get really fancy and buy costumes and elaborate craft supplies, you could easily drop a couple hundred. If you've got early literacy initiative grant money burning a hole in your cardigan pocket, go for it!

Day of Event

Step 1. Set up the room and prepare a clipboard with your liability and photo release waivers.

Step 2. Welcome patrons and briefly explain the format of the program. Lay out the standard ground rules (such as returning your mat/cushion when you hear the bell).

Step 3. Read or tell your chosen fairy tale and read its contemporary twisted version.

Step 4. Take this opportunity to have a little discussion that can lead to more mindfulness. Ask the kids which version of the story they prefer and why. Find out if they feel any sympathy for the antagonists in the fairy tales. Ask them, if they were going to act out the story (which they may do later if you are incorporating dramatic play) if they would prefer to be the hero or the villain in the story and why. Take this opportunity, if they'll allow it, to have a mini-discussion about "good" and "evil." For example, in *Ninja Red Riding Hood*, is the wolf really pure evil? Was he just hungry? Was he just doing what wolves do? What about at the end, when he stops eating meat? Is he now "good"? When stories are more ambiguous, like *Humpty Dumpty* and *After the Fall*, who is the "bad guy"? Was it Humpty, for having the accident? The wind? The wall? Who is the "good guy," the people who tried to put him back together again? How did Humpty feel about himself after he fell? Do stories have to have heroes and villains in order to be enjoyable?

Step 5. Do a few of the suggested yoga poses. Don't worry about being too formal.

Step 6. If you have costumes available, take this time for dramatic free play. Or, alternatively, do a craft related to the fairy tales. I'm sure you have lots of ideas in your storytime repertoire, but I've made some suggestions in the textbox on pages 60–61 to get you started.

Step 7. Ring the bell to signify the end of the program and ask everyone to help clean up.

Step 8. Say goodbye to your patrons and do the rest of the cleanup. Pat yourself on the back and take off your wolf ears!

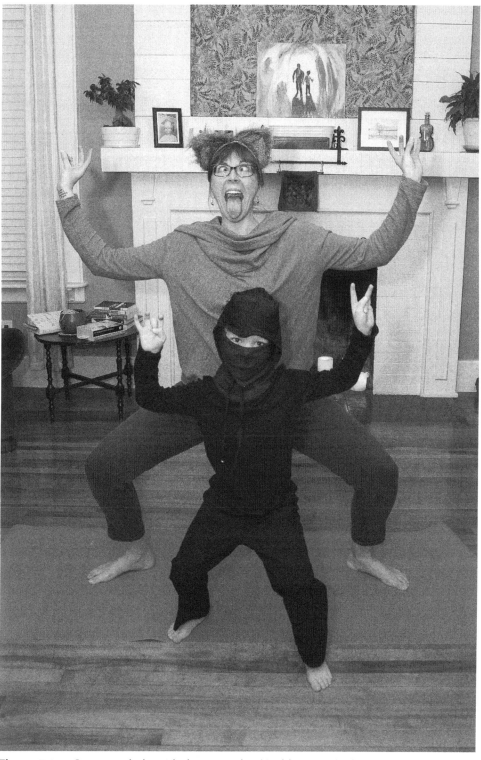

Figure 7.5. Costumes help with dramatic play (Goddess Pose). *Ebony Scott*

- For the mindful discussion part, you might only get to ask one or two questions (depending on the age range and size of your group) before everything dissolves into chaos. I consider that a win. Have reasonable expectations. This program model is written as a best-case scenario.
- Feel free to substitute any twisting yoga pose for the suggested poses since we are reading "twisted" fairy tales!
- Make sure to leave lots of time for free play at the end of the session so kids get time to act out the fairy tales or try out some yoga poses on their own.
- It isn't necessary to have yoga mats and props to deliver this program, but if you have them available it is a nice opportunity to introduce them and gets kids familiar with their many uses.
- Remember, sustained attention isn't a hallmark of this age group, so don't be surprised if they don't hold the poses very long or with much attention to detail. Don't worry about alignment at this point; focus on having fun.
- When the teacher wears a costume (wolf ears or a red cape, anyone?) it adds an extra element of enjoyment for the students and helps create a more immersive literary experience. This is the perfect time to bust out that martial arts uniform from your karate lessons!

SUGGESTIONS FOR CIRCULATING COLLECTION

The ABCs of Yoga for Kids by Teresa A Power and Kathleen Rietz.
Pacific Palisades, CA: Stafford House, 2009. ISBN 978-0-545-33955-1; Hardcover; Can$19.95.

This multi-award-winning and beautifully illustrated little book is a perfect combination of pre-literacy skill building and kinesthetic perfection! Aimed at preschoolers to early elementary, it lists the poses alphabetically with sweet drawings of children from different ethnicities practicing the poses in the shape of the poses' names (e.g., Flamingo has a little girl doing the pose next to a pink flamingo standing in the same shape). Each pose is explained through a singsongy rhyme, which is developmentally spot on for this age group. A must-have for every children's department, preschool, and elementary school library. Put it out on display near the play area and it won't last long.[10]

Animal Asanas: Yoga for Children by Leila Kadri Oostendorp and Elsa Mroziewicz Bahia.
New York: Prestel, 2017. ISBN 978-3-7913-7275-4; Hardcover; US$16.95/ Can$21.95.

This vividly illustrated hardcover has a colorful animal associated with each pose (includes the Sanskrit name) and a description of how to do the pose (mostly geared toward parents). There are helpful hints, such as "Tips for Parents with Lively Kids," a useful index at the end, and some wonderful relaxation mantras based on the colors of the rainbow. You could build a really great class out of these mantras by adding a few color/emotion-focused picture books, such as *My Many Colored Days* by Dr. Seuss or *The Color Monster: A Pop-Up Book of Feelings* by Anna Llenas. The book also comes with a splendid poster of the beautiful illustrations, which would look great in your children's department as a way to encourage movement. A must-have for every collection!

Breathe Like a Bear by Kira Willey and Anni Betts.
Emmaus, PA: Rodale Kids, 2017. ISBN 978-1-62336-883-8; Paperback; US$14.99/Can$17.50.

This adorably illustrated book is the perfect accompaniment to your children's programs, whether they are centered on yoga and meditation, or not. You can use the mini-mindfulness exercises to slip into other activities. For example, during a winter program do the "Hot Chocolate" exercise or "Rainstorm" on a rainy day. Also an excellent book to have on hand to recommend to parents and teachers who come to the reference desk looking for resources for children.

I Am Human: A Book of Empathy by Susan Verde and Peter H. Reynolds.
New York: Abrams, 2018. ISBN 978-1-4197-3165-5; Library binding; US$14.99/Can$18.99.

The third volume in Verde and Reynolds's I Am series, *I Am Human* focuses on our collective vulnerabilities and strengths. Our protagonist may be one in billions of people on this planet but that doesn't mean he isn't unique and that his path isn't equally important. Along the way he learns that using thoughtfulness leads to better choices and kindness can make bad things better. While humans are prone to making mistakes—to hurting and being hurt—that doesn't mean we can't ask for forgiveness or find common ground. And that should give us hope. The book ends with an author's note about how practicing loving-kindness meditation can improve emotional regulation and promote empathy. Verde offers children a sample meditation to try and detailed instructions, including how to offer loving-kindness to people who may be challenging, like a sibling or classmate. This colorfully illustrated book is simple and flashy enough to entertain preschoolers but deep enough to resonate with school-age children and even adults. An excellent addition to a juvenile circulating collection or to be used during storytime.

I Am Peace: A Book of Mindfulness by Susan Verde and Peter H. Reynolds.
New York: Abrams, 2017. ISBN 978-1-4197-2701-6; Hardcover; US$14.95/Can$17.95.

Our groovy protagonist may be covered in peace signs, but that doesn't stop him from worrying or feeling like a boat with no anchor. When this happens he takes a moment, finds his breath, and reminds himself that everything is all right. By feeling the ground under his feet, sharing kindness with others, talking about his feelings, connecting with nature, and using all his senses, he remembers that the only thing we really have is the here and now. This brings him peace. He declares, "I am PEACE." This simple book is a great tool to introduce the concepts

(continued)

of mindfulness to younger children. There's an author's note for parents explaining some of the science behind mindfulness and how teaching children these tools helps them strengthen their "attention muscle." Reynolds's rich, psychedelic illustrations add the perfect feel to yoga-teacher Verde's warm, concise text. The book concludes with a mindfulness exercise adults and children can practice together—imagining boats in our bellies—so fun!

I Am Yoga by Susan Verde and Peter H. Reynolds.
New York: Abrams Appleseed, 2015. ISBN 978-1-4197-2697-2; Board book; US$8.95/Can$10.95.

This colorful board book is the perfect introduction to yoga and mindfulness for your littlest patrons. Our protagonist tries to quiet her mind, still her wiggling body, and slow down her racing breath, but nothing works until she closes her eyes and says, "I am Yoga." When she is Yoga she can be tall like a tree, soar like a bird, dance with the moon, and stand up for herself (plus so much more). Each page is a beautiful watercolor wash of our girl trying each pose. By the end of the story she discovers that if she is Yoga, she is everything.

Mouse Was Mad by Linda Urban and Henry Cole.
New York: Sandpiper, 2009. ISBN 978-0-547-72750-9; Paperback; US$6.99.

This book gives no indication whatsoever that it is going to be about mindfulness and *Pranayama*. It sneaks up on you . . . like a mouse. And our mouse in this story is very, very angry. So angry he hops, stomps, screams, and rolls around in front of his friends. He just ends up dirty . . . and still mad. Until he gets standing-still mad. He stands perfectly still, takes deep breaths, and all of his friends join in. Until mouse realizes he's . . . not angry anymore. The staying still and breathing made him feel better, and all of his friends did too (not least because they no longer had to deal with a hopping-mad mouse!). A great book to use during preschool storytime to introduce some alternative methods for dealing with difficult emotions.

Stretch by Doreen Cronin and Scott Menchin.
New York: Atheneum, 2009. ISBN 978-1-4169-5341-8; Hardcover; US$15.99/Can$19.99.

Follow our doggy protagonist as he guides us through a variety of places and ways to stretch out our bodies. If you are nervous about teaching yoga to your storytime crowd, or think the word "yoga" may incite controversy in your library, this book is perfect. It delivers the same concepts as an introductory yoga picture book, but doesn't use any word other than "stretch" to describe it. While you're at it, check out the authors' other great physical literacy books: *Wiggle* (2005) and *Bounce* (2007). Cronin's website even offers activities to go along with the books.[11]

Yawning Yoga by Laurie Jordan and Diana Mayo.
San Francisco: Little Pickle Stories, 2017. ISBN 978-1-9397-7510-8; Hardcover; US$18.95.

This wonderful introduction to yoga may not be the best to use during storytime unless you are having a sleepover (all the poses center around going to bed), but it would make an excellent recommendation to give to parents with wired kids who need help winding down at night. It contains a comprehensive selection of poses with instructions, sweet little rhymes to go along with them, soothing illustrations, and even a glossary of terms and pronunciation guide. The author's interpretation of the traditional poses (calling *Jathara Parivartanasana* "Jelly Belly" and using it to help soothe worried tummies) is highly creative and also practical. You'll feel calm and sleepy just flipping through its pages. A must-have for collection development.

Yoga Bunny by Brian Russo.
New York: HarperCollins, 2017. ISBN 978-0-06-242952-0; Hardcover; US$17.99/Can$21.99.

Bunny wakes up one morning and starts his regular yoga routine. He invites Lizard to join him, but Lizard is too cranky; he invites Fox, but Fox is in a hurry; he invites Bird, but Bird has the hiccups. Bunny feels lonely that no one wants to practice with him, but he reminds himself that doing yoga alone is better than not doing it at all. As he starts Warrior Pose, some curious mice come by and decide to join him, soon all the other animals gather in the stretch session and discover it was exactly what they needed. This sweetly illustrated picture book does an excellent job reminding children (and adults!) that sometimes we need to be open minded to practicing something new and get out of our old routines and habits. The end papers contain lovely drawings of Bunny doing all the different poses. This book would be an excellent way to introduce yoga during a storytime, or a helpful story-pause during a kids' yoga class to remind everyone why it is important to keep practicing even if we have to do it on our own for a while.

You Are a Lion! And Other Fun Yoga Poses by Taeeun Yoo.
New York: Nancy Paulsen Books, 2012. ISBN 978-0-399-25602-8; Hardcover; US$17.99.

This endearing introduction-to-yoga picture book is perfect for ages two to four. It is illustrated with preschoolers from all different ethnic backgrounds in a garden practicing yoga together as the sun comes up. They do Lion, Dog, Butterfly, Snake, Frog, and many other poses (but not too many, just enough for short attention spans!). The instructions are easy to follow, and the drawings are adorable. If you are using the book during a preschool storytime, make sure to explain the meaning of the word *Namaste*, which features predominately in the story. Depending on the audience, I define the Sanskrit word *Namaste* as "My soul salutes your soul" or "All the good in me says hello to all the good in you."

SUGGESTIONS FOR PROFESSIONAL DEVELOPMENT COLLECTION

Little Book of Stars: 52 Relaxation Stories for Under 5s by Marneta Viegas.
Alresford, UK: Our Street Books, 2014. ISBN 978-1-78279-460-8; Paperback; US$14.95.

This sweet book is an excellent resource for adding mindfulness concepts to your preschool storytime programs or at the end of a Family Yoga Party during *Savasana*. Each little story involves a reflection, visualization, and breathing exercise that the children can follow along with as the adult reads in a soothing tone. You can pick a story based on that week's program theme; there are enough for an entire year in this little book! Watch over time to see if your regular visitors benefit from the calming moment in their day (you could even ask their caregivers for feedback). Some story examples are: Forgiving Star, Dancing Star, Magic Star, Truthful Star, and Safe Star. Also available as a box of fifty-two cards.

The Treasure in Your Heart: Stories and Yoga for Peaceful Children by Sydney Solis and Melanie Sumner.
Boulder, CO: Mythic Yoga Studio, 2007. ISBN 978-0-9777063-1-0; Paperback; US$19.95/Can$24.99.

First off, let me say with full disclosure that Sydney Solis is a dear friend of mine. But that said, I admired Sydney's work and admirable life story long before I had ever spoken with her. I first read this book when I was taking my children's yoga teacher training at Kripalu with Leah Kalish and fell in love with Sydney's approach to connecting to children through the physical *Asanas* and oral storytelling. Her books take single stories, chosen from a variety of cultural backgrounds, and pair them with a sequence of yoga poses, an activity, a chant or poem, and a meditation/visualization to create an entire lesson plan. Even if I don't follow the programs she has outlined, I often incorporate her carefully chosen and emotionally resonant tales into my children's (and adult!) yoga classes. The book contains photos of children from a variety of cultural backgrounds performing the *Asanas*, as well as a welcome appendix on how to use interfaith stories to teach in schools (or libraries). I would equally recommend her other book *Storytime Yoga: Teaching Yoga to Children through Story* (Mythic Yoga Studio, 2006), which I also use for programming.

Key Points

- When offering yoga and meditation to your youngest patrons, remember the key is to just give them a taste, not a full-on immersion, for which they do not have the attention span.
- Yoga and meditation programs for the early years can easily incorporate Every Child Ready to Read practices: writing, playing, singing, talking, and reading.
- When offering movement-based literacy programs to babies, most of it will be geared toward the caregivers, not the babies themselves.
- Program models for the age group can be easily adapted to fit into existing storytime formats or for use in outreach initiatives.

- Collection development of yoga and meditation materials for young children and their caregivers is important, and there are many books on the market available for both the general public and as resources for professional use.

Notes

1. Joseph Chilton Pearce, *Magical Child* (New York: Plume, 1992).

2. Shared Intelligence, *Library Rhyme Times and Maternal Mental Health—Action Research*, accessed November 16, 2018, https://sharedintelligence.net/our-work-2-2/library-rhyme-times -and-maternal-mental-health-action-research/.

3. Jane Dudman, "Books Are the Best Medicine: How Libraries Boost Our Wellbeing," *Guardian*, October 10, 2018, https://www.theguardian.com/society/2018/oct/10/books-best-med icine-how-libraries-boost-wellbeing.

4. Richard Fairgray and Jim Kraft, *Open in Case of Emergency* (New York: Sky Pony, 2017).

5. You can find good templates for making origami boxes online by Googling "origami box template."

6. Corey Rosen Schwartz and Dan Santat, *Ninja Red Riding Hood* (New York: Scholastic, 2015).

7. Bob Hartman and Tim Raglin, *The Wolf Who Cried Boy* (London: Puffin, 2004).

8. Aesop, "The Boy Who Cried Wolf," 1867 version, Lit2Go, accessed November 16, 2018, http://etc.usf.edu/lit2go/35/aesops-fables/375/the-boy-who-cried-wolf/.

9. Dan Santat, *After the Fall: How Humpty Dumpty Got Back Up Again* (New York: Roaring Brook, 2017).

10. A different version of this book review first appeared on www.yogainthelibrary.com.

11. Doreen Cronin, "*Wiggle, Bounce, Stretch*," DoreenCronin.com, accessed November 16, 2018, http://doreencronin.com/books/wiggle/.

CHAPTER 8

Yoga and Meditation for Elementary-Age Students

IN THIS CHAPTER

▷ Understanding the importance of offering yoga and meditation to elementary-age patrons

▷ Learning best practices for working with this specific age demographic

▷ Exploring three program models that can be modified to use in your library

▷ Discovering resources for your circulating collection and further professional development

---

Yoga and Meditation Programs for Children Aged Five to Eleven

AROUND THE TIME children begin school they are also learning how to separate from the family unit and make their way in the world. This shift continues into the preteen years, as friends' influences sometimes become more important than family traditions, and increases (often dramatically) by the time they become young adults. This precarious move toward independence is buffered by a strong connection to their teachers and other caregivers. Children who feel safer at home, accepted by their peers, and more connected in their communities experience this separation anxiety less.[1] Unfortunately, this is an ideal and not a reality for many of the children that come to our libraries' programs. As William Stixrud and Ned Johnson examine in *The Self-Driven Child: The Science and Sense of Giving Your Kids More Control over Their Lives,* when children feel like they have more internal locus of control, they experience less stress and are more intrinsically motivated to do their best.[2] Movement-based programs, especially ones that also incorporate mindfulness tools, really seem to help children with this quest for autonomy, something I've explored more rigorously in *Get Your Community Moving: Physical Literacy Programs for All Ages*.[3] Suffice it to say for our purposes here that presenting school-age children with opportunities at the library to learn coping skills that can benefit the rest of their lives is a win for everyone. Let's get started!

Program Models for Elementary-Age Children

These programs are designed for children who are old enough to be able to sit still for at least ten minutes at a time, so ideally those who have gone through preschool and perhaps even kindergarten, all the way through to age eleven or twelve. The next chapter explores programs for teens and young adults, but preteens (ages nine to twelve) may be comfortable attending classes from either chapter, so don't be too strict about age limits if your administration allows it. The first program model deals with using mindfulness techniques to handle letting go of things (including childhood) through the prop of a yellow balloon, plus engaging storytelling, and group sharing. The second program model invites families to follow their children's lead in an intergenerational yoga party! The last program gets even more physical literacy focused by adding movement into some mindful games that can be easily adaptable to the library, classroom, playground, or park.

Program Model: Bye-Bye Balloons

In this introductory mindfulness program designed for children aged five to ten (kindergarten to grade five), everyone gets to remember the experience of feelings of loss and

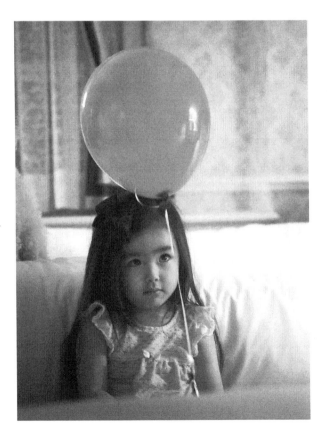

Figure 8.1. Balloons are fun and inexpensive props.

attachment from early childhood and share it with their older selves. By doing this, they get to look back on their younger selves with compassion and move forward by observing their own experiences in the present with a "wise mind." You will read *My Yellow Balloon* by Tiffany Papageorge (illustrated by Erwin Madrid), which tells the story of a young boy named Joey who gets a yellow balloon when he goes to the carnival.[4] The balloon man ties the yellow balloon's string to Joey's wrist, and from that day on Joey and his balloon are never apart. That is, until the string slips off his wrist and the yellow balloon floats away. Joey is devastated. He experiences all the emotions of grief: anger, confusion, sadness, longing, fantasizing it will return. His parents offer him comfort, and over time his sadness begins to fade and he thinks about the yellow balloon less and less. Then one day he sees a yellow orb in the water and runs to it, thinking his beloved has returned! But it is just the sun reflecting in the water. Instead of this making Joey sad, he realizes that whenever he sees the sun it can act as a reminder of his cherished balloon and then he will feel good again. The children get to experience this narrative emotional arc along with the younger Joey, promoting empathy and compassion, and everyone gets their own balloon tied to their wrist to practice being mindful with when they go home, as all their balloons will eventually pop, deflate, or float away.

Advance Planning

Step 1. Get a copy of *My Yellow Balloon* and read through it a few times to familiarize yourself with the story.

Step 2. Pick a day and time for the event. If you are in a school library, you can work with the teachers to secure a time; if you are in a public library, after school, evening, or weekends are probably best, unless you are creating it as a program for homeschool groups. You don't want the program to last longer than forty-five to sixty minutes, due to the relatively short attention spans of this mixed-age group (five to ten years old).

Step 3. Book the room you will be using. You'll need space for the kids and their guardians to sit comfortably and to run around afterward with their balloons. A quiet-ish space is best for the meditation part; the more you can minimize distractions, the better.

Step 4. Decide if it is going to be a drop-in or registration-only program. How many people can you accommodate in your space? How many kids can you (or your staff) handle?

Step 5. Make sure you have all the required materials (see list below).

Step 6. If this is a public event, advertise. Make a print poster. Make a Facebook event. Put it on your website and event calendar. Tweet about it. Share a teaser photo of a balloon on Instagram with details about the program. Visit local after-school centers and schools to drop off a poster for families to see.

Step 7. Do the paperwork. Make a sign-up sheet if you require registration. Prepare photo release waivers if you plan on taking photos/videos of the event.

Materials Required

- A copy of *My Yellow Balloon* by Tiffany Papageorge
- Cushions or chairs for seated meditation
- Yellow balloons filled with helium and attached to a ribbon or string
- Singing bowl or bell
- Sign-up sheets (if pre-registration is required) and photo/video release forms (if using)
- A watch, clock, or timer for keeping track of the meditation time

Budget Details

$30+. What sort of balloons and ribbon you buy will greatly impact the cost of this program, so work within your means. You are still a good person if you can't afford eco-friendly balloons. Costs can also be cut by buying a pack of yellow balloons at the dollar store and blowing them up yourself, but without the helium it won't be quite as magical. A hardcover copy of *My Yellow Balloon* is US$18.99, if you don't already have a copy in your system or attainable through interlibrary loan.

Day of Event

Step 1. Prepare the room by setting out the cushions and tying the balloons to a chair or coatrack. Get your photo release forms ready (if using).

Step 2. Greet your students and invite them to have a seat on one of the cushions and get comfortable. Once everyone has arrived, invite them to share their names and to guess what they think the balloons are for. Make sure any guardians are invited to join in.

Step 3. Do a few seated stretching exercises with them to get their fidgets out.[5]

Step 4. Read *My Yellow Balloon*, asking exploratory prompts as you go, and pausing to have everyone reflect on how Joey may be feeling in different parts of the story. At the end give everyone an opportunity to share a time when they were younger that they lost a special object. Ask them if there is anything (like the sun in the story) in their present life that reminds them of the lost object. If it is a large group, you'll have to remind the students to keep their answers short.

Step 5. Hand out the yellow balloons. Give the kids a few minutes to play with them and then ring the bell to bring them back to their cushions. If you don't give them time to interact with the balloons first it will be very hard for them to resist during the exercise.

Step 6. Have the students sit on their cushions and hold the balloon in front of them. Ask them to stare at the balloon and think about how they feel to be the owner of this yellow balloon. Then ask them to think about what will happen when the balloon deflates or gets lost or popped. Have them close their eyes and imagine the bright yellow sun and take deep breaths into their belly. Tell them that if feelings of sadness or anger come up with the thoughts of losing their balloons that that is OK, it is perfectly normal. Have them bring their attention back to their sun images and take nice deep breaths. Ask them to open their eyes and stare at their balloons and take nice deep breaths. Have them give their balloon a hug and say, "I appreciate you, balloon. I know that when we have to say goodbye I will remember you whenever I see the sun." Have them let go of the balloon (still hanging on to the string) and watch the balloon float toward the ceiling (assuming you filled the balloons with helium). They can say, "Goodbye, balloon" if they'd like. Have them close their eyes and take deep breaths and notice how it feels to let go of their balloons. Hold this space for two full minutes (or more; gauge your audience). Ring the bell and have them open their eyes.

Step 7. Thank them all for coming and ask if anyone would like to share their experience of what it was like practicing letting go of the balloon. Thank everyone for sharing; then ring the bell and give them free time to play with their balloons before their parents/guardians or teachers arrive. Expect a few pops and possibly tears (depending on the ages). Use this as an opportunity to practice with the breath and for everyone to show empathy for their friend who lost their balloon.

Advice

- Children have a short attention span. Adults too. Don't take it personally if they all don't love meditation or sitting still the first (or tenth) time. Don't expect too much. Try not to show disappointment or impatience with them if they fidget. Lead by example; perhaps they will follow.
- This program works best with five to ten students, but can be done with a larger class; you just may want to skip the sharing portion. You can offer paper and pencils/markers at the end for students to draw their experience with a special object.
- Keep praise general; do not single any one child out for "sitting still" or "focusing." Emphasize the non-competitive nature of meditation. For some it will be harder than others.
- Use plain language and simple instructions, especially with the youngest children.
- Use a gentle and soft tone of voice, but not singsongy or syrupy. You are not telling lullabies. Be alert, but not rushed, as you read the story and do the mindfulness exercise afterward.
- It is always better to have too many balloons than not enough. I recommend pre-registration for this program to make sure you don't run out.
- I prefer biodegradable natural latex balloons and cotton twine, which are twice the price but better for the environment.[6] Work within your budget.
- Stress to children (and caregivers) that even if you bought eco-friendly balloons they shouldn't be released into the sky because they can damage birds and other wildlife.
- Be careful to get the right book. There are a few children's books on the market with similar titles, such as *The Yellow Balloon*, **One** *Yellow Balloon*, and **The Big** *Yellow Balloon*. You want **My** *Yellow Balloon* by Papageorge and Madrid (though I'm sure those other titles are lovely too!).
- Consider building a book display of other books that are about children and their special objects. Here are some suggestions to get you started: *Elmer and the Lost Teddy* by David McKee, *Knuffle Bunny* by Mo Willems, *Llama Llama Time to Share* by Anna Dewdney, *Kiki's Blanket* by Janie Bynum, *Owen* by Kevin Henkes, and *Dad and the Dinosaur* by Gennifer Choldenko.
- Any of the above books could replace the balloon theme and be done with teddies, blankies, and so forth instead, but the ephemeral nature of the balloon makes it especially poignant. Flowers or other delicate objects would also work well. If the program is a success, consider offering it multiple times with different themes and titles.
- Don't assume older kids don't still have attachment objects and won't identify with Joey (even if they won't admit it). I know grown adults who can't sleep without their special pillow or teddy bear!
- This program could also be shortened to thirty minutes and modified for preschool storytime; just make sure to add some movement and keep the meditation portion super short—two minutes at most!
- With older kids (ages eight plus) you could try purposefully popping the balloons and practicing with the loss in real time. You may or may not want to offer replacement balloons to take home. I would recommend letting the students know at the very beginning as you give them their balloons that they will be popping them.
- Feel free to add some upbeat music to the free-play session at the end. To encourage pattern recognition, see if they can bounce their balloons along with the beat.

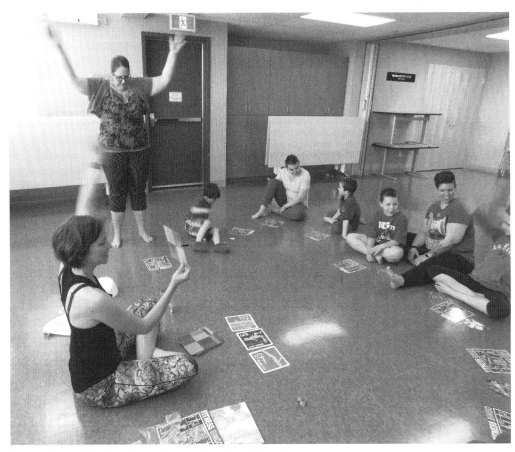

Figure 8.2. Playing fitness bingo. *Brendan Helmuth*

Invite patrons to bring their family and friends for this intergenerational yoga party. Designed to have the kids lead some of the program, it is a great opportunity to empower elementary school–age children to model healthy behavior for their younger siblings and parents or other family members. Yoga is truly for everyone! The class starts out with some warm-up games and poses; then the kids take turns teaching from a deck of yoga cards; then there is a yoga-related story, some games or free play, and even a healthy snack!

Advanced Planning

Step 1. Decide who is going to run the program. Do you feel comfortable leading children and adults through some simple yoga poses, or would you rather hire a professional yoga teacher (if you don't already have one on staff)? Find a yoga teacher in your community, if you need one. Bonus points if they will volunteer to teach for free! Familiarize yourself with the sequence on page 78.

Step 2. Decide how long the program will be. Our Family Yoga Parties are sixty minutes (forty-five minutes of yoga and fifteen minutes of coloring or free play at the end).

Step 3. Determine if it will require pre-registration and what the age parameters are. If you are marketing it as a family program (but it is mostly geared toward elementary-age students), do you want babies to be able to come? Grandparents? My answer is always

"Yes, the more, the merrier!" but you might not feel the same way. If you are giving everyone a healthy snack, how many can you afford to feed?

Step 4. Pick a time, date, and location (in consultation with the yoga teacher, if you are hiring one). Book the room.

Step 5. Gather all necessary supplies (see list below).

Step 6. Prepare liability waivers, photo/video releases (if using) and sign-up sheet (if you require pre-registration).

Step 7. Advertise your event. Make a fun poster and share with local schools, recreation centers, day cares, and anywhere else you usually post. Make a shareable Facebook event and also post to other social media accounts.

Materials Required

- A deck of yoga cards (there are some great suggestions in chapter 5)
- Yoga mats, block, and straps
- Beanbags
- Music, if using, and something to play it on
- Singing bowl or bell
- Necessary paperwork (waivers)
- Yoga-related book for storytime (suggestions: *The Happiest Tree: A Yoga Story* by Uma Krishnaswami and Ruth Jeyaveeran or *My Daddy Is a Pretzel: Yoga for Parents and Kids* by Baron Baptiste and Sophie Fatus, and there are many more listed at the end of this chapter)
- Physical literacy games/props, like fitness bingo or fitness dice (if using)
- A healthy snack (see the "Advice" section below for suggestions)
- Coloring sheets (if using)

Budget Details

$20–$100+. If you already have all the mats and props (beanbags, music, bell, fitness items), then you'll just need to buy the snack supplies, which, depending on how many attend the program and what you serve, could run from $20 to $100, or more. You'll also need to pick up a yoga card deck ($15) and one of the suggested books (hopefully you already have something in your collection). You'll also need to find funding to pay for a yoga teacher if you aren't leading the class yourself or couldn't source a volunteer. There may be wellness or fitness grants available to cover this; don't be afraid to ask for money!

Day of Event

Step 1. Prepare your healthy snack. Cut up vegetables; get out the blender or juicer, or the napkins, or whatever else you might need. Don't forget a garbage can or compost bin!

Step 2. Prepare the room for your party and welcome the yoga teacher, if you hired one. Go over the plan for the program.

Step 3. Welcome your patrons and have them complete the necessary waivers.

Step 4. Follow along with the infographic on page 78, adapting as necessary.

Step 5. Wrap up the program and thank everyone for coming. Solicit feedback from parents and kids, if appropriate.

Family Yoga Party

Jenn Carson is a physical literacy expert, yoga instructor, librarian, and the author of *Get Your Community Moving: Physical Literacy Programs for All Ages.*

This intergenerational program is designed for all ages and abilities to have fun together increasing their physical literacy skills through yoga, storytelling, mindful games, and healthy nutrition. The sequence involves lots of transitions to keep busy bodies moving and engaged!

1. Bean Bag Balance (a) From lying down, balance a bean bag on one foot, then pass to the other foot, then pass from foot to hand and then hand to hand. (b) Balance the beanbag on the head and then come into standing. (c) Take turns passing beanbags onto the heads of people who have dropped their beanbag. Notice how height differences can add to the challenge!

2. Head to Knee Pose From seated position, place right foot along left thigh, twist heart over left knee, and reach toward left foot with the hands. Hold for 5 breaths. For an added challenge, place the right foot across the left thigh and reach behind the back with the right hand, grasping the left big toe. Fold towards left knee. Repeat on left side.

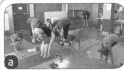 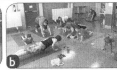
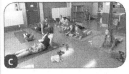 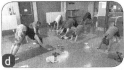

3. Sun Salutation (a) Reach arms overhead. Fold over toward toes and then lift halfway. (b) Plant hands on the ground and step feet back into a Plank (push-up) Pose. (c) Lower to the ground, lift chest, and look up. (d) Lower head and push back into Down Dog (inverted V shape). Look forward and step feet between hands, reach hands overhead and lower hands to heart. Repeat whole sequence 3-5 times.

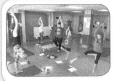

4. Tree Pose Turn right foot to a 90° angle. Lift right foot to calf or inner thigh. Bring hands in Prayer Pose to the center of chest. Option to raise arms overhead. Take 5 breaths. Lower the foot and repeat on the other side.

5. Cat/Cow Pose (a) From a kneeling position, place both hands on the floor, shoulder-width apart. Inhale and look toward the ceiling. (b) Exhale and arch the back upward, tucking the chin. Repeat both poses 9 more times.

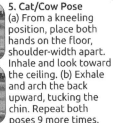

6. Dancer Pose (a) From a standing position, externally rotate the right shoulder and grasp the inside of the right foot. Reach the left hand in the air. (b) Leaning forward, push the right foot into the hand, arching the back slightly and balance. Hold for 5 breaths and switch sides.

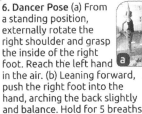 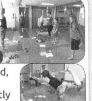

7. Yoga Card Deck Grab a deck of yoga cards and have each student pick one. Take turns and one by one have a student demonstrate the pose they chose and then lead the class in following along. If someone doesn't want to play "teacher", that's OK.

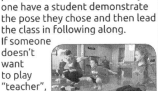

8. Yoga Hug After the game, everyone can give themselves a hug for being brave and teaching class. They can also give their family members and friends hugs if they'd like.

9. Storytime Read a story about yoga or meditation and follow along with the poses or exercises in the book. *The Happiest Tree: A Yoga Story* or *My Daddy is a Pretzel: Yoga for Parents and Kids* are good choices.

10. Physical Literacy Game Play a game of fitness bingo, roll fitness dice, or play games from a mindfulness or yoga card deck. Or play tag, hide and seek, or other classic schoolyard games.

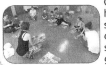

11. Healthy Nutrition Break Make fresh juice, if you have access to a juicer. Or smoothies, if you have a blender. Or simply enjoy some pre-cut fruit and vegetables.

12. Free Play Put out some fitness related props (balls, blocks, pogo sticks, stilts, jump ropes, Frisbees, mini-bowling sets, binoculars, empty cardboard boxes, hula hoops, balloons, etc...) and let kids and adults play.

13. Prizes Send everyone home with some cool party swag. Many physical literacy non-profits like Active for Life will supply prizes like these t-shirts. Or buy some bouncy balls or glow sticks at a dollar store. Or give out yoga-pose coloring sheets.

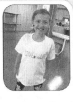

www.jenncarson.com • www.yogainthelibrary.com • www.physicalliteracyinthelibrary.com

Figure 8.3.

Advice

- Make sure to follow your state or provincial laws regarding proper food handling safety when preparing the healthy snack. Anyone in my library who prepares food to serve the public must have completed a food safety handling course that is recognized by the provincial government. Check with your administration about your local regulations. Be especially mindful if the children are going to help with the preparation.
- Here are some healthy snack ideas that have worked for me in the past: fresh juice or smoothies, carrot sticks and other cut-up veggies, cut-up watermelon (especially popular in the summer), real-fruit popsicles, fruit leather and nut-free granola bars, applesauce, apples, oranges, and bananas (cut in half), crackers and cheddar/marble cheese, brown bread and butter, yogurt tubes, veggie chips, pita and hummus.
- Fitness dice, fitness bingo, and other physical literacy games can be easily sourced online with a quick Google search. If you are short on prep time or funds, play an old-fashioned game like hide-and-seek, tag, dodgeball (use a very soft ball!), or Simon says. They are classics for a reason.
- Feel free to add music during free play at the end of the session. I caution against using it during the instructional time, as it can be distracting. Singing songs or dancing together is always a fun idea!
- Be brave and consider telling an oral story rather than reading a picture book. Sydney Solis has some amazing yoga-related stories and poses that accompany them in *The Treasure in Your Heart: Stories and Yoga for Peaceful Children* and *Storytime Yoga: Teaching Yoga to Children through Story*.[7]

Program Model: Mindful Games

Rather than having a formal class focusing directly on meditation, sometimes the best way to teach mindfulness techniques to elementary-age children is by playing games and

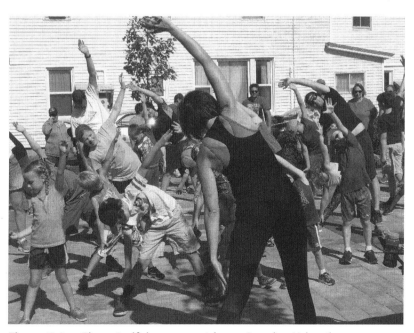

Figure 8.4. Play mindful games outdoors. *Brendan Helmuth*

having fun. This way they learn skills that can directly translate to their daily lives when they play at home or school, by themselves or with friends. This program model includes a variety of games that can be offered in separate sessions, or you can pick and choose a few favorites for a one-off program. They can also be modified to suit students with limited mobility or other exceptionalities. The games can be added into existing library programs, be a stand-alone session, or (for school librarians and teachers) they can be used in the classroom as mindful breaks.

Advanced Planning

Step 1. First you'll need to decide who is going to run the program and whether it is going to be a one-off event or a recurring program. Decide how long the program will be. Thirty to forty-five minutes is probably plenty, shorter if you are using the games as a "break" from another activity. Will it require pre-registration? What are the age parameters? Are you willing to open it up to younger/older siblings or parents/guardians and make it an intergenerational program?

Step 2. Pick a time, date(s), and location. Book the room.

Step 3. Read through the list of games below and choose which ones to include. It is always good to have a few extras in hand in case one of them isn't going over as planned or doesn't take as long as you thought it would. Play the games yourself (grab a co-worker if necessary) to get a better understanding of what you'll be asking the kids to do. Walking incredibly slowly is much harder than it sounds!

MINDFUL GAMES

- Art Stations: Set up multiple mindful art stations where children can silently work on free-form projects with no end goal. The key is to keep the space process oriented, and that way there is no need to ask questions about how to make it look "right" or feel like there is a goal or someplace they need to "get to" in the art-making process. Put out paper, scissors, glue, pens, pencil crayons, card stock, stickers, and so forth and let them make whatever they'd like. Have different stations in the room with different supplies or color themes.
- Beanbag Toss: Have children stand in pairs facing each other, about three feet apart. Tell them to concentrate on throwing the beanbag as accurately and gently as possible to their partner. Ask them to notice the feeling as it leaves their hands, watch it fly through the air, and notice the feeling when they catch it. Ask them to watch their breath during the process. Then have them all take one step backward and repeat. Have them keep doing this until they are so far apart they can't throw accurately anymore (or else you run out of room). A great game to play outdoors as well.
- Moving Meditation: Gather students in a large room, gymnasium, or a green space/deserted parking lot. Tell them you are going to play a game where the objective is to walk as slowly as possible, like a slow-motion scene from a movie. Have them form a line and walk in a circle, one following the other. Ask them to notice if they get frustrated that the person in front

of them is going too slow and see if they can challenge themselves to walk even slower. As they are walking, ask them to notice which part of their foot hits the ground first, how their knee flexes and bends, how their arms and shoulders move when they walk, and which part of their foot is the last to lift off as they step forward. As the children become more adept at this, switch up the game to have them walk sideways or backward, or vary the speed (fast, medium, slow), or vary the length of each step (giant steps, baby steps, etc.). You can also have them try concentrating on other movements, such as hopping, skipping, or slow jogging. If you are in a gym that has lines on the floor, or a park or playground with sidewalks or trails, have them follow a linear path without touching the sides, roots, rocks, or the cracks.

- Bell Game: Have children walk mindfully around your space, and then randomly ring a bell or singing bowl and have them freeze in place and listen to the bell. When they can no longer hear its vibration (and only then!), they can begin moving again. Repeat. Perhaps allow everyone a turn as the "bell ringer."

- Big Breaths in Small Spaces: If your library doesn't have a large activity room or access to a green space, you can do movement-based mindfulness programs in small spaces. In a small public space, like a corner of the children's department, a study room, in between the stacks, or a hallway, try playing balancing games like standing on tiptoes and trying to reach for the ceiling or the top of a shelf. Or do standing yoga poses that involve balancing, like Tree Pose. Ask the children to notice what happens to their breath and their bodies as they reach high. Then have them duck down and crouch into little balls and notice their breath and how their lungs and bodies feel all scrunched up. Take a ride in the elevator and tell everyone to try holding their breath as they go to the top floor. Then go back down again and have everyone notice their breath flowing in and out of their nostrils. Have children practice walking up and down the library's stairs or front steps mindfully: holding the rail, taking one step at a time, watching the step ahead of them, and so forth. Form a train and have them follow you through the library, being extra quiet, like mice in a conga line. Have them try to follow lines on the carpet or jump quietly from floor tile to floor tile on their tiptoes. Have older children spread out and see if they can find their own quiet breathing space in the library—a little nook they can curl up in—and challenge them to take ten deep breaths in that space and then come back to your meeting spot to report on the place they found and what made it special to them.

- Take a Walk: Have children create imaginary rivers using scrap fabric, blankets, or towels and jump from one imaginary rock or bank to another (these could be pillows, beanbags, or construction paper cutouts of rocks . . . or just totally imaginary). Hide plastic insects, butterflies, fish, or animals along the folds of the fabric or throughout the play space that students can find (but must leave in their place for the next person to discover!). Afterward have everyone sit quietly and read a good book together about rivers or nature walks, such as *I Took a Walk* by Henry Cole, *A Walk in the Forest* by Maria Dek, or *There's a Barnyard in My Backyard* by David Suzuki.

Step 4. Gather all required materials (see list below).

Step 5. It is always a good idea to have a liability waiver for any movement-based programs in case someone gets hurt. Consider if you also want photo/video releases. Prepare a sign-up sheet (if using).

Step 6. Advertise. Make a print poster (if you do that sort of thing) and/or add to your calendar of events. Put it up on social media (Facebook, Twitter, Instagram). If you have a YouTube channel, make a little teaser video of someone doing one of the games. Share it with local elementary schools, sports clubs, Scouting groups (there's got to be a badge for this!), and so forth.

Materials Required

- Art supplies: paint, pom-poms, glue, stickers, pencil crayons, markers, paper, tape, cardstock, scissors, and so on. The sky's the limit here!
- Beanbags
- Bell or singing bowl
- Yards of scrap fabric, towels, or blankets
- Plastic insects, fish, animals, and so forth
- Liability waivers, photo/video releases
- A book about walking mindfully, such as *I Took a Walk* by Henry Cole or *There's a Barnyard in My Bedroom* by David Suzuki or *A Walk in the Forest* by Maria Dek

Budget Details

$15–$200+. Depending on which games you choose and what props you already have on hand, this could be a fairly low-cost program requiring little more than a trip to the dollar store for a few packages of plastic insects or fish. If you have to buy a bunch of art supplies, plus a book, plus beanbags and a singing bowl, you are going to run closer to $200 or more, depending on how many students you have.

Day of Event

Step 1. Gather all required materials. Set up the room or space according to whatever games you intend on playing.

Step 2. Welcome everyone to the program and have parents/guardians sign the paperwork.

Step 3. Play the games! Have all the fun!

Step 4. Have kids pitch in to help clean up after games. Use this as another mindfulness game. Talk about how you can mindfully put art supplies or toys away. Have them follow their breath and really pay attention to the texture and color of everything they are touching: the wooden handle of the paintbrush, the bumpy feel of the beanbag, and so forth. Challenge them to try this at home when they are cleaning up their rooms, brushing their teeth, or washing dishes.

Step 5. Gather everyone in a circle while you wait for parents/guardians to pick them up and ask them their favorite part of the program. Ask them what they found the most challenging. Pass a beanbag around to encourage turn-taking and remind interrupters that only the person with a beanbag may speak and that this is a good opportunity to practice their listening skills.

Advice

- Give as many opportunities for free play and self-directed learning as possible during the games. If the children offer suggestions of different ways to play, be willing to try them out. Allow "rules" to be modified. Create the space for mindfulness and then let them explore it. You will be surprised what you may learn. The most unassuming Zen masters are often small children. They catch small details that we distracted, controlling adults often miss.

- There is value in "dangerous" play. If children are balancing or hopping on ledges or railings while doing their walking meditation, as long as they are not excessively high, consider letting them. There are many books and studies on the value of letting children take small physical risks that demonstrate it actually improves their ability to concentrate and greatly increases physical dexterity.[8]

- When planning the program, consider opening it up to a large age range. When children are allowed to play with kids older or younger than them, it puts them in the zone of proximal development, where they can learn skills from someone more skilled than them that they couldn't learn alone or with peers their own age. For example, during the free-play art activities, if younger children sit next to older ones, the older children can offer suggestions and provide inspiration, as well as help by opening paint tube caps or demonstrating a difficult technique. Or during the beanbag toss, pairing an older child with a younger one will require the older ones to pay close attention and adapt their throwing to the developing skill set of the younger players. This helps deepen the mindfulness aspect of the play, as the elder child must concentrate on their movements to help the younger one, and the younger one must follow closely the elder's lead so they can keep up. The less you, as the facilitator, interfere the better. This interaction is just as beneficial for the older students, as it allows them to practice patience and empathy and they improve their skills through teaching.

- There are many materials on the market that offer mindful game ideas. Check out *Mindful Games Activity Cards: 55 Fun Ways to Share Mindfulness with Kids and Teens* by Susan Kaiser Greenland and Annaka Harris (which I review in chapter 5) or *Mindful Movements: Ten Exercises for Well-Being* by Thich Nhat Hanh and Wietske Vriezen. There are also more resources listed in the collection development textboxes below.

SUGGESTIONS FOR CIRCULATING COLLECTION

50 Ways to Feel Happy by Vanessa King, Val Payne, and Peter Harper. Lake Forest, CA: QEB Publishing, 2018. ISBN 978-1-68297-311-0; Hardcover; US$14.95/Can$19.95.

Vanessa King is a positive psychologist and the author of the evidence-based book for adults, *10 Keys to Happier Living* (Headline, 2017), which she's now adapted for a younger audience. This colorful book is chock full of great activities and ideas to get kids thinking about such important things as how to connect with others, how to bounce back after a setback, and how to take care of their bodies.

(continued)

There are also important sections on what to do if the reader feels unhappy and how to incorporate more mindfulness into one's day through taking a "mindful minute" or a "mindful walk," or having a "mindful snack." A great resource to share with patrons aged seven to twelve.

A Handful of Quiet: Happiness in Four Pebbles by Thich Nhat Hanh.
Berkeley, CA: Plum Blossom Books, 2012. ISBN 978-1-937006-21-1; Spiral-bound hardcover; US$14.95.

This sweet little book is full of practical ways for parents or guardians to share mindfulness with the children in their lives. It includes a pebble meditation, a drawing meditation, craft ideas, a song, and a list of further resources. A lovely addition to your circulating collection and for use during programs.

The Happiest Tree: A Yoga Story by Uma Krishnaswami and Ruth Jeyaveeran.
New York: Lee & Low, 2005. ISBN 978-1-60060-360-0; Paperback; US$8.95.

This award-winning story follows young Meena while her class puts on their very own interpretation of *Red Riding Hood*. Meena is worried she is far too clumsy to take any part in the play, but her teacher insists on assigning her a role as a tree. Meena is very concerned about this and expresses her fears to her parents, who try to reassure her. She goes to the Indian grocery store with her mother and sees a yoga class practicing in the back room. She is invited to join the children's class but refuses for fear of being too clumsy. She eventually joins anyway and finds with time, practice, and attention she gets better at keeping her balance, both on and off the mat. In fact, she uses her special yoga breathing to stay calm when something goes wrong the night of the performance. The story ends with a little explanation about yoga's origins and some drawings of Meena doing different poses. The best part of Krishnaswami's writing is how it weaves Meena's Indian culture and her mother tongue into the text, grounding the reader into the history of yoga and bringing its heritage alive. An excellent picture book to use for yoga storytime or recommending to patrons.

My Daddy Is a Pretzel: Yoga for Parents and Kids by Baron Baptiste and Sophie Fatus.
Cambridge, MA: Barefoot Books, 2004. ISBN 978-1-8414-8151-7; Hardcover; US$16.99.

The plot behind this picture book is that in a yoga class the teacher asks all the kids to name what their parents do, and our protagonist says how his daddy can do that too. So someone says how their mom is a gardener and he says, "Sometimes, my daddy's a tree." Then on the next page it shows how to do Tree Pose with illustrations and instructions. The next child says their parents are vets and our narrator says, "Sometimes, my daddy's a dog." Then on the next page it shows how to do Dog Pose. It continues on like this for nine poses. A nice little introductory text about yoga for kids, it is also available in a deck of fifty cards called *Yoga Pretzels: 50 Fun Yoga Activities for Kids & Grownups* (US$14.99), which are great for passive programming or yoga storytimes.

Play Yoga: Have Fun and Grow Healthy and Happy! by Lorena Pajalunga and Anna Láng.
Milan, Italy: White Star Kids, 2017. ISBN 978-88-544-1111-1; Hardcover; US$14.95/Can$16.95.

While there are many books on the market to introduce parents and young children to yoga, one this colorful and engaging deserves mention. Especially since it focuses on yoga as a "game" and the author reminds parents not to hold poses for very long or expect children to be able to stay still. Instead she encourages adults to respect these bodies in constant growth and transformation and urges readers to play at inventing stories with the characters of the book: the lion, the seagull, the crocodile, the yak, and many others. The illustrations by Láng feature plump, rosy-cheeked children and their serene-looking animal counterparts. Though there is an effort at gender balance among the children, it is disappointing that they are all fair skinned. A little more diversity among the characters would have been more appealing.

Yoga for Kids and Their Grown-Ups: 100+ Fun Yoga and Mindfulness Activities to Practice Together by Katherine Priore Ghannam and Tanya Emelyanova.
Emeryville, CA: Rockridge Press, 2018. ISBN 978-1-93975-489-9; Paperback; US$15.99/Can$20.99.

Broken into chapters, including sequences and a visual library of poses, and including an index of yoga activities, this is a workhorse of a book for parents, teachers, or curious kids and a definite must-add to your collection (both professional and circulating). There are also chapters on empowering kids through yoga, family yoga time, yoga games (including storytimes!), meditations, and partner poses. Written in accessible language, the author makes special mention of how yoga can benefit those on the autism spectrum or with ADHD, and includes safety tips for concerned parents. Aimed at children aged three to twelve and their caregivers, you can tell this book was written by a former public elementary school teacher, the tone (perfectly matched by Emelyanova's illustrations) is so soothing and inviting, anyone would want to try yoga!

Yoga for You: Feel Calmer, Stronger, Happier! By Rebecca Rissman.
Lake Forest, CA: Walter Foster, Jr., 2017. ISBN 978-1-63322-319-6; Hardcover; US$14.95/Can$19.95.

This helpful introductory yoga instruction manual is aimed at the eight-plus age group. We have it classified as juvenile in my branch, but it would be right at home in a young adult collection as well. There's a brief history of yoga and introduction to mindfulness, meditation, and *Pranayama*, and it even broaches the "Is yoga a religion?" subject. There is a brief description of many of the more popular styles of yoga, and it talks about how to choose a class that's right for you (which may be a little beyond the grasp of kids who are still learning to ride their bikes). The book is divided into two sequences: one for "energizing" and one for "calming," but the poses can also be practiced on their own. While this book has some solid theory in it, and is an excellent introduction to the topic, my major beef is that the illustrations are very feminized and this may turn off some kids who don't identify as cis-gendered female. A few less hearts, flowers, and ponytails could go a long way to making the book more accessible, but if you have the budget, I would still add it to your collection and use in displays.

SUGGESTIONS FOR PROFESSIONAL DEVELOPMENT COLLECTION

How to Teach Meditation to Children: Help Kids Deal with Shyness and Anxiety and Be More Focused, Creative and Self-Confident by David Fontana and Ingrid Slack. London: Watkins, 2017. ISBN 978-1-78678-087-4; Paperback; US$16.95/ Can$18.95.

Now in its third edition, this classic teaching manual has meditations designed for children aged five to eight, nine to twelve, and thirteen to eighteen, making it an excellent resource for public or school librarians dealing with multiple age demographics. I particularly like the authors' approach to secular meditation, which is the same approach I feel we should take in libraries. They offer a "word of warning" that though parents and teachers may be concerned that due to kids' impressionable natures by introducing meditation we may be indoctrinating them with Buddhist principles, this is unfounded. The Buddha was just a person who tried to systematically understand, practice, and share the practice of meditation. A religion was built up after him. They urge practitioners to avoid too much visual imagery or "flights of meaningless fantasy" and to instead ground the practice in the breath and mindfulness. There are a great many exercises to explore mindfulness and more concentrated periods of meditation with all these age groups. Highly recommended.

Meditate with Me: A Step-by-Step Mindfulness Journey by Mariam Gates and Margarita Surnaite.
New York: Dial Books, 2017. ISBN 978-0-399-18661-5; Hardcover; US$17.99.

This is my go-to book to use for teaching meditation to kids aged five to ten. In fact, this book is like a ready-made program. Buy it immediately! Even if you've never done a moment of meditation before in your life, you can read this book with the kids and have them make "glitter bottles" out of recycled bottles with glitter, water, and food coloring, just like in the story. Another craft idea is to have them paste cotton balls on a blue paper sky to make the "thought clouds." They can add lightning or sunshine or whatever else they might be feeling that day. The book features cheerful animals learning how to be aware of their breath, their feelings, and the world around them. There is a four-step meditation process included at the end of the book, which parents may find helpful as well.[9]

Once upon a Pose: A Guide to Yoga Adventure Stories for Children by Donna Freeman. Victoria, BC: Trafford, 2009. ISBN 978-1-4269-2220-6; Paperback; Can$22.77.

This unique book of ten yoga adventure stories take twenty to forty minutes each and are designed for children aged three to twelve. The best part? They are in French and English—perfect for presenting bilingual programs in a province like New Brunswick, Ontario, or Quebec, and extremely useful for teachers in the French immersion programs of the Canadian school system. There are 108 classroom applications for preschool to grade six, along with modifications for exceptionalities such as autism, ADHD, cerebral palsy, Down's syndrome, and asthma, making yoga accessible to everyone. Each *Asana* is explained and accompanied with a black-and-white photograph and its French and Sanskrit title. The book includes a helpful letter to parents (or skeptical naysayers) that you can use as a template detailing the benefits of the library's yoga programs. This book is one of a kind; be sure to add it to your collection and also use it when planning programs.[10]

Yoga for Children: 200+ Yoga Poses, Breathing Exercises, and Meditations for Healthier, Happier, More Resilient Children by Lisa Flynn.
Avon, MA: Adams Media, 2013. ISBN 978-1-4405-5463-6; Paperback; US$17.95/Can$18.99.

Written by a mom and yoga educator, Flynn knows firsthand the difficulty of helping kids self-regulate. At age six, her son was diagnosed with ADD and sensory processing disorder. While this book is mostly geared toward helping parents facilitate yoga sessions with their children, it is a necessary and thorough resource for all children's yoga teachers. Supported with scientific research that lists the benefits of yoga for children (increased balance, strengthened immune system, improved sports performance, enhanced listening skills, and much more!) and brings the results into the library/classroom. Turns out yoga also encourages community, improves executive functioning, and helps increase confidence instead of competitiveness. Flynn stresses that yoga has been proven to aid speech development "through slow, repetitive verbal instructions, songs, and the imitation of simple sounds found in nature." She considers breath work (*Pranayama*) for speech development essential, because we speak on the exhale, so the more breath support we have, the more chance for expression. Flynn breaks her instructions down by developmental age group (two to four, four to six, seven to ten, ten to twelve), which is perfect for the library educator planning yoga programming sessions for children. With sections on individual *Asanas*, sequences, massage, partner poses, breath work, games, songs/chants, and visualization, this manual really is the "bible" of children's yoga instruction and is absolute required reading for anyone interested in teaching yoga to children and preteens, whether you are a parent or professional.[11]

Yoga for You & Your Child: The Step-by-Step Guide to Enjoying Yoga with Children of All Ages by Mark Singleton.
London: Watkins, 2016. 2nd edition. ISBN 978-1780288758; Paperback; US$14.95/Can$15.95.

So many yoga books, especially those geared toward kids/parents, have a proprietary bent: they are trying to sell you on the author's "brand" of yoga or want you to take their teacher training. Mark Singleton is not one of these yoga merchants. He cut his teeth teaching yoga to disadvantaged children in India and then returned to the UK to teach in schools and after-school centers. It shows in the delivery of his book with its straightforward tone, its clear instructions, and refreshingly plain-clothed models (sweat pants and T-shirts for everyone!). Besides sections of simply named poses, there are also games and dynamic movements. Male and female caregivers are doing the poses alongside the children. There's a great section reminding parents/caregivers of the importance of having their own yoga practice before trying to instruct their children, so they can act as a good role model and embody the yogic philosophy in their daily actions. Although some teachers disagree with teaching *Pranayama* (breathing exercises) to children,

(*continued*)

Singleton has a thorough introduction to the topic with some practices tailored to little lungs. The same is provided for meditation. There is a section called "Putting It All Together" that links the *Asanas* into a series you can practice at different times (when you or your child is sluggish, or hyper, or recovering from an illness, for example). And most useful is a section at the back called "Yogis at School" that uses yoga philosophy to help children cope with the stresses of school, to improve their concentration, and even how to write exams "the yoga way." Highly recommended for all public and school libraries, including professional collections for libraries that host yoga programs.[12]

⚛ Key Points

- When offering yoga and meditation to school-age children, remember to work with their limited attention spans, reinforce a non-competitive atmosphere, and focus on having fun and giving them skills that breed resiliency.
- This age group spans a wide range of development. Program models can be adapted to meet the needs of the children participating and to work with changing environments, such as doing outreach in a park or playground.
- Incorporating multimodal literacy components into these programs is easy when there are so many elements present in each program model: movement, free play, writing/drawing opportunities, storytelling and sharing, dramatic play, reading, and music.
- Collection development of yoga and meditation materials for school-age children and their caregivers is important, and there are many resources on the market available for both the general public and as resources for professional use.

⚛ Notes

1. Carla Hannaford, *Playing in the Unified Field: Raising & Becoming Conscious, Creative Human Beings* (Salt Lake City, UT: Great River Books, 2010).

2. William Stixrud and Ned Johnson, *The Self-Driven Child: The Science and Sense of Giving Your Kids More Control over Their Lives* (New York: Viking, 2018).

3. Jenn Carson, *Get Your Community Moving: Physical Literacy Programs for All Ages* (Chicago: ALA Editions, 2018).

4. Tiffany Papageorge and Erwin Madrid, *My Yellow Balloon* (San Francisco: Minoan Moon, 2014).

5. Check out video resources at www.yogainthelibrary.com for examples.

6. These can easily be ordered online and taken to your local party store to be filled with helium.

7. Sydney Solis and Melanie Sumner, *The Treasure in Your Heart: Stories and Yoga for Peaceful Children* (Boulder, CO: Mythic Yoga Studio, 2007) and Sydney Solis and Michele Trapani, *Storytime Yoga: Teaching Yoga to Children through Story* (Boulder, CO: Mythic Yoga Studio, 2006).

8. For example, Angela J. Hanscom, *Balanced and Barefoot: How Unrestricted Outdoor Play Makes for Strong, Confident, and Capable Children* (Oakland, CA: New Harbinger, 2016).

9. A different version of this book review first appeared on www.yogainthelibrary.com.

10. A different version of this book review first appeared on www.yogainthelibrary.com.

11. A different version of this book review first appeared on www.yogainthelibrary.com.

12. A different version of this book review first appeared on www.yogainthelibrary.com.

Yoga and Meditation for Teens and Young Adults

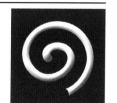

Yoga and Meditation Programs for Teens and Young Adults

DEANE JUHAN HAS WRITTEN the most apt description of the way teens carry themselves that I have ever read in *Job's Body: A Handbook for Bodywork*. He calls them "tightly wound springs" whose muscular tension is a result of mental and physical turmoil that builds up as they navigate the uncertain territory of impending adulthood.[1] Young adulthood is a time of change. Changing friends, changing opinions, changing bodies, changing interests, and even changing identities. Meditation and yoga have been proven in small-scale scientific trials to reduce mental health issues, such as anxiety, in teens; so why not offer classes for free at the library?[2] Teens and twenty-somethings are one of our hardest-to-reach demographics, so anything we can do to draw them into the building (while also helping them feel awesome!) is worth a shot.

Program Models for Teens and Young Adults

To grab the attention of overscheduled or socially isolated young adults, we need to get creative. We have to think about what their needs are: social connection, no-cost programs, stress reduction, self-care, healthy coping skills, exercise, positive body image, and so forth. And we also need to think about their vast and ever-changing interests (pop culture, music, art, sports, video games, anime, relationships, cars, food, etc.) and how we can entice them to get their needs met while entertaining them with subject matter that intrigues them. The first program model, Rhythm & Flow Yoga for Teens (see below), is a yoga sequence set to live music. Our library offers this class for teens and adults, and it is extremely well attended. The second program model, Stress Less for Teens (page 96), uses meditation, journaling, and small behavioral changes to help teens find some inner calm. Both these programs touch on multimodal forms of literacy (music, writing, reading, playing, storytelling, physical literacy, etc.) and therefore appeal to different types of learners with different strengths and abilities.

◎ Program Model: Rhythm & Flow Yoga for Teens

Teens have an overwhelming amount of stress in their lives, something we adults sometimes forget or overlook as we rush about our busy days grumbling about our adult responsibilities. On top of that, they are often acutely self-conscious of their bodies, and getting them to participate in a yoga class in front of their peers can sometimes prove difficult. A great way to loosen them up and help them overcome their shyness is to include live music in the class. Here in Woodstock we've had a multi-instrumentalist and several extraordinary guitarists grace our classes over the years. Our most popular guitarist plays a lot of groovy funk on an electric guitar. If you can't find a local musician, have some teens you know help you create a rad playlist of music they love.

Advance Planning

Step 1. Pick a time and date for the program. After school, evenings, or weekends are best for teens (unless you are in a school library and can offer it at noon). Keep in mind that many have after-school or summer jobs and busy social lives, so don't plan for more than an hour-long class.

Step 2. Book the room you'll be using.

Step 3. Decide whether the class is going to be a one-hit wonder or a regular weekly or monthly event. You could try it and if you get a good response, book more sessions. You'll also need to decide whether it is going to be a drop-in or pre-register session.

Step 4. Secure a yoga teacher if you aren't planning on teaching the class yourself. Local yoga studios may have teachers willing to volunteer their time, especially if they get to promote their studio and classes to teens. Some teens may have more discretionary spending than most people realize, especially in affluent neighborhoods. This could be a selling point for a teacher. But if you are qualified to teach, I highly recommend it—it's a super fun sequence!

Step 5. Find a local musician to play during the class. While it might be tempting to recruit another teen to play, that might cause the students to be distracted by their peer's presence. Also, a teen might not have the experience and repertoire to be able to play for a full hour unless the teen is a classically trained musician. It doesn't hurt to give them an audition first! You are looking for someone who can play music (no singing, unless is it quiet chanting) relatively non-stop for an entire hour and can vary the tempo of the music to correspond to the teacher's instructional arc. I recommend meeting with the musician beforehand and going over your plan for the class and what sort of music you'll require them to play at what times (slow and calming for *Savasana*, rhythmic and engaging for *Vinyasa* work). Some top choices for instruments would be acoustic or electric guitar, cello, flute, piano, harmonium, or kora. If you can't find anyone suitable, you can create a playlist of teen-approved music instead.

Step 6. Gather all necessary resources (see "Materials Required" section below).

Step 7. Prepare your paperwork (liability waivers, sign-up sheets, photo release forms, etc.). You may also want to print off copies of the routine to hand out so students can practice at home, or provide them with a digital link.[3] Consider administering a short evaluation form at the end to gauge how your audience felt. They may not readily volunteer information publicly but may be more willing to share anonymously in an online survey or paper form.

Step 8. Familiarize yourself with the yoga sequence (see pages 92–94) or discuss with your hired instructor what they will be teaching.

Step 9. Advertise the event. Make sure to share to places teens go: Instagram, Snapchat, YouTube, Twitter, Facebook, the mall, sports clubs, coffee shops, the high school, and so forth. You'd also be surprised how many listen to the local radio in their cars, so it wouldn't be a bad idea to do a public service announcement or call in to a morning show to plug the program.

Step 10. Secure funding to pay for the teacher/musician, if required.

Step 11. Make a display of yoga-related material to refer patrons to after class.

Materials Required

- Mats, blocks, and straps for all participants (you may also want a few chairs handy for patrons with limited mobility in case you need to make modifications)
- Singing bowl or bell
- Liability waivers, photo release forms, evaluation forms, and other handouts
- Chair or meditation cushion for musician and music stand, if required
- Consent cards
- A water bottle—this sequence is going to get you sweating!

Budget Details

$0–$500+. If you already have all the yoga props, can find a teacher and musician to volunteer for the class, and provide digital links to handouts, this could be a relatively no-cost program. On the other hand, it could go in the opposite direction if you hire a pricey musician and teacher and have to buy all the props from scratch. In my experience, it falls somewhere in the middle range. I teach the classes myself, and if I have a musician who volunteers their time I still buy them some sort of thank-you present: a gift certificate to a local restaurant, a locally made piece of pottery, a bouquet of flowers, or potted plant. Or I pay the musician between $50 and $100 per hour, depending on their level of experience. Either way, you should do something to let them know their time and effort is valuable to you. Remember, they had to practice the songs, bring their own equipment (sometimes renting things!), and travel to your library. The same applies if you are hiring a yoga teacher (especially if they are bringing their own mats and props). Grants may be available through local art, music, and wellness organizations. The cost to print out the take-home yoga sequence on nice glossy sheets at your local print shop should be about $30 (depending on how many you get done).

Rhythm & Flow YOGA for TEENS

Teens have stress too! Grab a friend and a yoga mat, or shut your bedroom door and rock out alone. Put on some jams that soothe your soul and try out these poses. No need to do them all, or do them perfectly, just give it a shot! Extra credit challenge: turn off your phone while practicing.

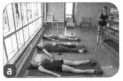

1. Opening *Savasana* (a) Lie on your back with a beanbag, book, or phone on your belly. Roll your feet out to the side and turn your palms up to face the ceiling. Take a deep breath and feel your belly lifting toward the ceiling. As you exhale, lower your belly button toward your spine. Repeat 5 times. (b) Point and flex your toes 5 times.

4. Standing Forward Bend (a) Reach forward and hook your big toes with the first two fingers of each hand, fold upper body over your legs. Take 5 breaths. (b) Lift your feet and place the palms of your hands under the soles of your feet, fold over your legs. Take 5 breaths.

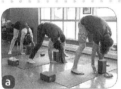

9. Open V Forward Bend (a) Step your right foot to the back of your mat and turn toward the right, facing the long side of your mat. Bending at the waist, lower your head toward the ground, placing your hands on the ground. Take 5 breaths and then come back up slowly. (b) Option to place block under your head for support, or rest the head on the floor.

2. Mountain Pose Come into standing with your feet hip width apart. Lift your toes and lower them slowly, feeling the floor solid under your feet. Lift your heart toward the ceiling. Relax your shoulders. Relax your jaw. Take 5 breaths.

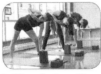

5. Triangle Pose Step your right foot back. Place your left hand on your left thigh, the floor, or a block/book, and twist your torso toward the right. Take 5 breaths. Repeat on the left side.

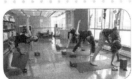

10. Open V Forward Bend Twist Return to pose #9, but this time place your right hand on the floor or a block, and twist the body to the left, with left hand raised in the air. Lower your left hand and place it on the floor, lift your right hand, twisting to the right. Repeat 4 more times on each side.

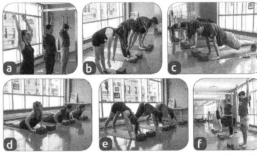

3. Sun Salutation (a) Reach your arms overhead. (b) Fold over toward your toes and then lift halfway. (c) Plant your hands on the ground and step your feet back into a plank (push-up) position. (d) Lower to the ground, lift your chest and look up. (e) Lower your head and push back into Down Dog position (inverted V shape). (f) Look forward and step your feet between your hands, reach your hands overhead and lower your hands to your heart. Repeat whole sequence 3-5 times.

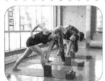

6. Reverse Triangle Step your right foot back. Place your right hand on your left thigh (or the floor/block) and twist toward the left. Take 5 breaths. Repeat on the other side.

7. Side Angle Pose Step your right foot back. Bend your left knee and place your left elbow on it. Twist your torso toward the right and reach your right arm overhead. Take 5 breaths. Repeat on the left side.

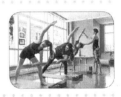

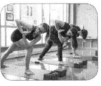

8. Reverse Side Angle Step your right foot back. Bend your left knee and reach your right elbow over your left knee. Twist to the left. Bring your hands to heart center. Take 5 breaths. Repeat on the other side.

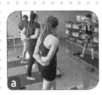

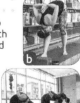

11. Pyramid Pose (a) Step your right foot back. Reach behind your back and hold your opposite wrists or elbows. (b) If you have the shoulder flexibility, place your hands in reverse prayer behind your back. (c) Bend over your left knee, twisting slightly toward the left. Take 5 breaths. Repeat on the other side.

Figure 9.1.

Rhythm & Flow Yoga for Teens

12. Tree Pose (a) Turn your right foot to a 90° angle. (b) Lift your right foot to your calf. Bring your hands in prayer pose to the center of your chest. (c) Option to lift foot to inner thigh and raise arms overhead. Take 5 breaths. Lower the foot and repeat on the other side.

13. Down Dog From Mountain Pose, bend over and place your hands on the floor next to your feet. Step your feet to the back of your mat and lift your hips in the air, creating an inverted V shape. Line up your ears with your arms and tuck your chin. Take 5 deep breaths.

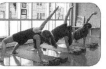

14. Flipped Dog From Down Dog, lift your right leg in the air and bend your knee. Drop your right foot to the ground on the left side of your mat, flipping your chest toward the ceiling and reaching the right arm overhead. Take 5 breaths. Come back to Down Dog. Repeat on the left side.

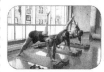

15. Side Plank Come into Plank Pose (push-up position) and roll onto the right side of your right foot, stacking your left foot on top and turning your torso to the left. Lift the left arm in the air. Hold for 5 breaths. Roll back to Plank and repeat on the other side.

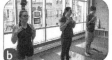

16. Body Tapping (a) Standing in Mountain Pose, lightly tap your left arm with your right hand, then tap your right arm with your left hand. (b) Tap your chest and belly. (c) Tap your hips and legs. (d) Tap your feet, the back of your legs, your bottom, lower back, mid-back, upper back (or whatever you can reach!), shoulders, back of the head, top of the head, and (gently!) your face.

17. Toe Squat with Shoulder Stretch (a) Sit on your heels with your toes tucked under. Grasping the end of a strap, reach your right arm overhead and let the strap dangle down your back. Reach behind your back and hold the other end of the strap with your left hand. Bring the hands as close together behind the back as possible. (b) Option to clasp fingers in gable grip instead of using strap. Hold for 5 breaths and repeat on left side.

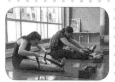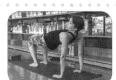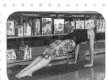

18. Seated Forward Bend Sitting with your legs out in front of you, wrap the strap around the soles of the feet. Walk your fingers down the strap, coming closer to your toes. Hold the elbows out to the side. Take 5 deep breaths.

19. Reverse Table Top Plant your feet flat on the floor and place your hands on the floor behind you, with your fingers facing your feet. Lift your hips off the ground toward the ceiling, flattening your torso. Option to let the head fall back if that feels good for your neck. Hold for 5 breaths, then lower.

20. Slide Pose Reach your legs out long in front of you and place your hands on the floor behind you, with your fingers facing your feet. Lift your hips off the ground toward the ceiling, flattening your torso and keeping your legs as straight as possible. Try to touch your toes to the mat. Option to let the head fall back if that feels good for your neck. Hold for 5 breaths, then lower.

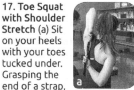

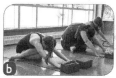

21. Shoelace Pose (a) Place your right foot by your left sit bone. Cross the left leg on top, trying to stack the left knee on top of the right. (b) If possible, lean forward over the knees. Hold for 5 breaths. Repeat on the other side.

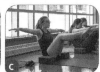

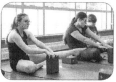

22. Boat Pose (a) Rock back and balance on your bottom, lifting your bent knees in the air and holding underneath them. Hold for 5 breaths. Lower legs. (b) **Uplifting Pose** Cross ankles, place hands on blocks next to hips, lift bottom off the ground. Hold for 5 breaths. Lower. (c) Repeat Boat Pose, this time letting go of the knees and stretching the arms to the side. Lower legs. (d) Repeat Uplifting Pose. (e) Repeat Boat Pose, this time straightening the legs.

23. Leg Lift Place right foot in by left sit bone. Lift left leg, holding on to block for support. Point toes and make 3 clockwise circles, then 3 counterclockwise circles with entire leg. Lower left leg. Repeat on right side.

www.jenncarson.com • www.yogainthelibrary.com • www.physicalliteracyinthelibrary.com

Figure 9.2.

Rhythm & Flow Yoga for Teens

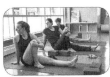

24. Seated Twist From seated position with your legs out in front on you, bend your right knee and place your foot on the ground near your right sit bone. Wrap your left hand around your right thigh and place your right on the floor behind you. Exhale and look over your right shoulder. Hold for 5 breaths. Repeat on the left side.

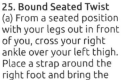
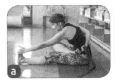
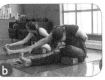

25. Bound Seated Twist (a) From a seated position with your legs out in front of you, cross your right ankle over your left thigh. Place a strap around the right foot and bring the strap behind your back, grabbing it with your right hand. Lean forward and hold your left foot or toes with your left hand (or rest the hand on your leg). (b) Option to place a block under the bent knee for support. Hold for 5 breaths. Repeat on the other side.

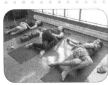

26. Twisted Roots Lie on your back and place your feet flat on the floor. Walk your feet and your hips to the right side of your mat, leaving your torso and head in the middle. Cross your right knee over your left and drop your knees to the left. Place your left hand on your right thigh (the one on top) and take your right arm out at a "T" shape to the side. Hold for 5 breaths. Repeat on the other side.

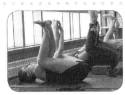

27. Happy Baby Lie on your back with your feet in the air and your knees bent. Reach between your legs and wrap your hands around the outside of your feet or ankles. Lower your knees toward the ground and take 5 deep breaths.

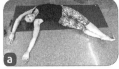
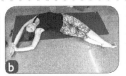
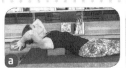
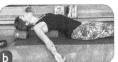

28. Banana Pose (a) Lie on your back and walk your feet and arms to the right. (b) Hold your left wrist with your right hand and pull gently. Cross your left ankle over your right ankle. Take 5 breaths. Repeat on the left side.

29. Modified Fish Pose (a) Lie on your back with one block between your shoulder blades (option to use a bolster or rolled up mat if this is too intense). (b) Place another block underneath your head. Arms come out to the side in a "T" shape and palms roll up toward the ceiling. (c) Option to place the head directly on the floor for a more intense neck stretch.

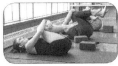

30. Self-hug Bring your knees to your belly and wrap your arms around your knees. Give your legs a gentle squeeze. Rock from side to side to give your lower back a slight massage. Take 5 deep breaths.

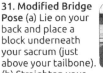
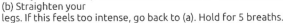
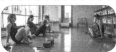

31. Modified Bridge Pose (a) Lie on your back and place a block underneath your sacrum (just above your tailbone). (b) Straighten your legs. If this feels too intense, go back to (a). Hold for 5 breaths.

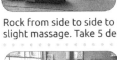

32. Bound Forward Bend From an easy sitting position (or Lotus or Half-Lotus) reach behind your back and hold your opposite elbows or wrists. Inhale and look toward the ceiling. Exhale and fold your torso over your knees. Lower your head to the mat or a block, if possible. Hold for 5 breaths.

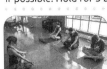

33. Meditation Pose Sitting in an easy cross-legged position (or Lotus or Half-Lotus) place the back of your wrists on the fronts of your knees. Tuck your index finger under your thumb. Straighten the other three fingers toward the floor. Tuck your chin and close your eyes, or gaze softly in front of you. Hold for 10 breaths.

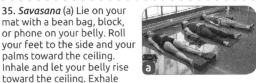
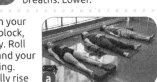

34. Uplifting Pose Cross ankles, place your hands on the blocks or mat next to hips, lift your bottom off the ground. Hold for 5 breaths. Lower.

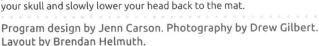

35. *Savasana* (a) Lie on your mat with a bean bag, block, or phone on your belly. Roll your feet to the side and your palms toward the ceiling. Inhale and let your belly rise toward the ceiling. Exhale and lower your belly. Close your eyes and continue this relaxing breathing for at least 5 minutes. Stay as long as you like. (b) Have a partner place their hands around your feet and give a gentle squeeze to the arch of your foot with their thumb. (c) Have a partner gently cradle your head in their hands while they apply mild pressure at the base of your skull and slowly lower your head back to the mat.

Program design by Jenn Carson. Photography by Drew Gilbert. Layout by Brendan Helmuth.

Figure 9.3.

Day of Event

Step 1. Welcome your musician (and yoga teacher if you aren't leading class yourself). Help them set up and prepare the room for students to arrive.

Step 2. Greet students at the door and have them sign their waivers/release forms (or their parents/guardians if they are underage).

Step 3. Once everyone is settled, welcome them and thank them for coming. Acknowledge that for some of them it might be their first time trying yoga and that they are very brave for showing up. Remind them not to worry about what anyone else is doing on their mats, to just focus on their own bodies and their own practices. Remind them that yoga is about having a conversation with ourselves and about learning who we really are.

Step 4. Follow along with the yoga sequence outlined in the infographic on pages 92–94, modifying as necessary for those with injuries or mobility issues.

Step 5. After you ring the bell to bring everyone out of *Savasana*, thank them for coming to class, suggest they stop by the stacks to check out the yoga books and DVDs (bonus points if you made a display ahead of time!), and hand out the infographics (if you printed them) to take home to practice the sequence on their own. If this is a recurring class, remind them of the next session and the date and time. Don't forget to give your musician a round of applause! Hand out evaluation forms, if using.

Step 6. Clean up and go record those stats!

Advice

- Try to meet with the musician ahead of time to figure out the tempo for the class and make sure they can follow along with your transitions. You want to make sure

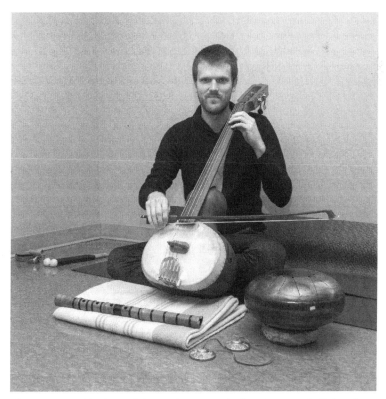

Figure 9.4. Find musicians whose music fits the mood of the class.
Brendan Helmuth

the music suits the mood of the program. Ask them what you can do to help them feel most at ease while playing and set them up in a space that works best for them.

- You have the choice whether you set up the room ahead of time, putting out all the mats and props, or letting the students choose their own mat and where to put it down. If size constraints are an issue because your room is small or you are expecting a lot of people, setting up the mats ahead of class allows for optimal spacing and saves time as everyone is arriving. If you have a smaller crowd or lots of space, give students the chance to select their own mats and props and land wherever they feel comfortable in the room. A little bit of autonomy sometimes goes a long way with this age group.

- Teens will be nervous, chatty, and incredibly self-conscious in front of each other. Ignore their outbursts, flirting, and giggles and just keep teaching. Show them how to follow the breath and focus on the pose. Lead by example. They will, in time, quiet down. For some of them, it might take a few sessions. Remember, for those who are most self-conscious, blithe humor or cynicism is a smokescreen for their discomfort. Have empathy but also set strong boundaries for the sake of everyone participating. If you need to ask someone to take a break because they are really disrupting the class, I would frame it like this: "Hey, you seem to be having a hard time staying on task here; would you like to take a five-minute break and come back and join us when you've settled down, or would you like to keep going?" Only use when absolutely necessary.

- Don't be afraid to do hands-on assists with teens, as long as you (and they) are comfortable. Provide consent cards so they know they have the choice whether to be touched or not. Make sure they know they can change their mind at any point during the practice. When talking about assists at the beginning of class you open the door to an excellent opportunity to have a mini-discussion about consent. Explain to the class what the assists are for, when you might be doing them, and the best way for them to let you know whether or not touch is welcome. Explain that consent is an essential part of any touch, including non-sexual touch. This gives the teens an excellent opportunity to practice deciding whether they want to be touched and expressing it, and also that it is OK to change their mind.

◉ Program Model: Stress Less for Teens

After years of teaching yoga to teens and twenty-somethings, I developed this program after stumbling upon the book *Be Mindful & Stress Less* by Gina M. Biegel.[4] I assumed it was a book written for adults based on the title and was planning to review it for my website, but once I skimmed through the first few pages I realized it was aimed at teens and it was brilliant! Teens and college-age kids are, in my experience as a public librarian, one of the hardest demographics to reach for mindfulness-based programs. I've had more luck when I ran programs in a university environment or high school, because I was going to where my audience was already hanging out all day long. But getting reluctant (and oh-so-busy!) young adult patrons into my public library had always been difficult. So I came up with this short after-school program to get the conversation going with students in my community. I sent them home with Biegel's book so they could explore and practice the techniques we flirted with on their own time and in the privacy of their own spaces.

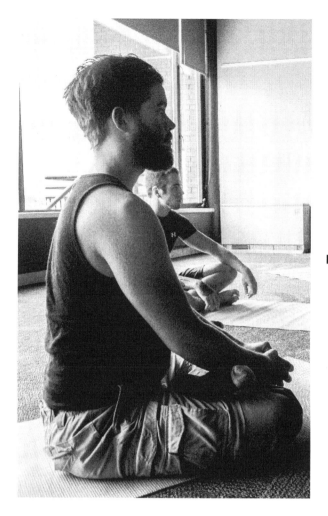

Figure 9.5. Teens can enjoy meditation. *Drew Gilbert*

This book could be a lifeline to a stressed-out student—it is something I certainly wish I had when I was that age—and getting copies into clammy, anxious hands is a step in the right direction to improving young adult mental health.

Advance Planning

Step 1. Decide who is going to facilitate the program (preferably a staff member with experience with meditation) and when you are going to offer it. I'd recommend after school or evening. Teens can be very busy on the weekends, though that is an option too. If you work in a high school library or university/college library, you could offer it as a lunch 'n' learn program. If offered at a public library, consider age restrictions. Our library offers it for thirteen- to nineteen-year-olds, but you do what works for your audience. Some of the topics discussed might not be appropriate for preteens, and a very large age range may result in less shared experience among participants and may hinder dialogue.

Step 2. Pick a date and book the room. I've offered this as a one-off program, just to whet their appetites for mindfulness and send them home with a book to learn more. But it could easily be turned into a series of programs, following along with Biegel's activities in the book or from her comprehensive website.[5] The best space is a room with few distractions and out of the public eye, so the participants are more likely to feel comfortable sharing.

Step 3. I recommend making this a registration-required event, since you will need to order books ahead of time (unless that is out of your budget; look under "Budget Details" and "Advice" for alternative ideas). Five to ten is a good number of students, so everyone has enough time to share, if they want to, but the group is big enough that no one feels obligated to talk if they don't want to. Prepare a sign-up sheet.

Step 4. Advertise the event. Share on social media, create a print poster, add it to your calendar of events, and put it on your website. Most importantly, share it with the adults who are most aware of the students who would benefit from the program. Make sure those teachers, coaches, guidance counselors, and parents/guardians have the opportunity to encourage teens to show up by giving them lots of advance notice and details of the program.

Step 5. Get a copy of *Be Mindful & Stress Less* and read through it. Pick out a few activities to try with the students. In the "Day of Event" section below I've picked out my favorites.

Step 6. Secure funding for the books and order them well in advance so they arrive in time.

Step 7. Gather all other materials listed below.

Materials Required

- Enough copies of *Be Mindful & Stress Less* by Gina M. Biegel for everyone to take home, or at least one copy for you to work from
- Chairs and tables to sit at
- Scrap paper and pencils/pens or else blank notebooks
- A singing bowl or bell or app on your phone
- A healthy snack (nut-free granola bars, for example)

Budget Details

$15–$200+. The list price for Biegel's book is US$14.95, so if you buy at least one book to use as a guide for the program and skip the snack, that's the most cost-effective approach. You could essentially even just get exercises off her website and do the program for absolutely no cost, but as libraries, it is important to support authors and the reading of books, right? If you can apply for a wellness grant (which is what I did) to cover the cost of the books, use free journals donated by a local non-profit, and buy a box of granola bars and a pack of juice boxes, you'll also be putting this on for a song. If you've got tons of cash you need to spend, feel free to go all out.

Day of Event

Step 1. Set up the tables and chairs and put out the snacks. Teens will be hungry, especially if you are offering this after school.

Step 2. Welcome everyone to the group as they arrive. Explain the format: they will be learning some different activities that can help with stress relief. They are free to get up and use the bathroom or have a snack whenever they want. Ask them to please turn off their phones or set to airplane mode. There are pencils/pens and paper to write down their thoughts during the exercises. They have the opportunity to share if they want, but it is optional. Then go around the table and ask everyone to say their name, what grade they are in, and one thing that they do to relax and one thing that causes them stress.

Step 3. Set the tone by having them take a moment of mindfulness before you begin. Ask them to sit up straight in their chairs and feel their feet flat on the floor. Ask them to place their hands in their laps and feel their fingers resting on their thighs. Ask them to close their eyes and feel the cool air as it enters their nostrils and the warm air as it leaves. Have them notice the breath coming in and going out. Let them breathe silently for a few more breaths, and then ring the bell and ask them to open their eyes. Explain that this exercise was a mini-example of meditation. Ask them to share if it felt hard or easy to sit silently. Ask them how they felt when the bell rang.

Step 4. Choose a few exercises from Biegel's book. The number will depend on how much time you have and how many students attend; the more students, the longer the sharing portion will take. Here are the ones I've used with success: #18 Mindful Hobby: Use Info, #20 Mindful Downtime, #21 Mindful Calling, #22 Look Up from Your Device, #23 Self-Care, #47 It Is So Silent in Here. Read the section, and when it comes to a question have them jot down their answers in their notebook or on the scrap paper. If everyone has their own books, you can take turns reading out loud. Allow time for asking questions and for sharing their answers, if they feel comfortable.

Step 5. As you finish the last exercise, encourage the teens to take their books home with them and make a commitment to reading one of the fifty sections every day. Ask them to mark the date on the calendar and in two months see if their stress levels have dropped any from integrating some of the practices in the book into their lives.

Step 6. Hand out evaluation forms and thank everyone for coming.

Advice

- Resist the urge to swear. Especially if they are swearing, because swearing is super contagious. If you, like me, have the mouth of a sailor, you may find the urge to curse creeping up on you in the presence of almost adults. For some reason the middle-aged adult brain subconsciously thinks swearing in front of teens will gain their acceptance and make you look cooler. Those are lies! Resist! Be professional!

- If you cannot raise the funds to purchase the books, no matter how hard you try (or your audience is just too big), consider making a "cheat sheet" handout of your top three or four techniques from the book that students can take home with them. Or, as an alternative, if you can get funding for collection development, buy numerous copies and students can check them out or place them on hold.

- Whether you can afford to give out the books or not, be sure to share Gina M. Biegel's web page of resources for teens: https://www.stressedteens.com/resources-for-teens/. It is full of great (downloadable and printable!) activities and tip sheets such as "Mindful Messaging and Posting Practice" or "10 Ways to Minimize School Stress." You could even build a whole program around these simple but effective tip sheets and activities if you didn't have time to read the book (or access to a copy).

SUGGESTIONS FOR CIRCULATING COLLECTION

Be Mindful & Stress Less by Gina M. Biegel.
Boulder, CO: Shambhala, 2018. ISBN 978-1-61180-494-2; Paperback; US$14.95/Can$19.95.

I'm a firm believer that every young adult should take a course on mindfulness-based stress reduction as part of their high school curriculum. And if that just isn't feasible, then they should at least get a seminar and a copy of this book. If you can't convince the school district to offer it, why not host one at the library? (See page 96, "Stress Less for Teens.") There are many smart exercises in this book, such as speaking in M-I messages (mindfully checking in and then using "I" statements to express how you feel) or doing a fundamental needs assessment, which you can use to easily build a self-reflective, accessible program that teens really relate to—and be grateful for the road map to navigating the tricky, often painful waters of adolescence. The author even offers an appendix with special recommendations for people experiencing a variety of issues such as autism spectrum disorder, depression, vision loss, anger, self-harm, or addiction to social media. If nothing else, buy a copy for every teenager you love and for your young adult collection.

Breathe: Yoga for Teens by Mary K. Chryssicas.
New York: DK Pub, 2007. ISBN 978-0-7566-2661-7; Book & DVD; US$14.99/Can$17.99.

This reasonably priced, colorful, and creative book with accompanying DVD is perfectly geared toward teens. Featuring photographs of real teens from various ethnic backgrounds doing yoga poses and including inspiring quotes from celebrities, it is very easy for teens to feel that these exercises and yoga tenets are accessible, easy to read, and fashionable. I do wish the publisher would have included male models and/or models of varying body size. The book opens with a brief history of yoga, breath work, and *Chakras*, and then gets right into the poses with attention-grabbing names like "hip-hop hips," "lightning bolt," and "hero's twist" and then an inspiring series of practices with names like "wake-up call" (for the morning), "bendy back," and "yoga booty." There is also a section on self-care and suggestions for what to do "if you're not flexible," "if you have a headache," or "if you have back problems." This is a decent resource for teens; my only concern is the obvious gender bias and focus on weight and appearances (such as a section of poses you can do "if you're overweight" featuring very thin models). There is also a cheesy spiritual undertone to the manual that reflects the author's own beliefs (like referring to "radiant angels" for guidance). Despite its flaws, I still consider this a worthy addition to any circulating collection and especially appropriate to have out on display during teen yoga programs.[6]

Mindfulness for Teens with ADHD: A Skill-Building Workbook to Help You Focus & Succeed by Debra Burdick.
Oakland, CA: Instant Help Books, 2017. ISBN 978-1-62625-625-5; Paperback; US$17.95/Can$24.95.

This workbook is useful to have on hand for teens or parents requesting resources to help themselves or their child who is struggling with ADHD. The book offers some excellent mindfulness-based exercises that may be alternatives or used in conjunction with more traditional treatment for the disorder. Includes helpful chapters on how to deal with part-time employment, driving, sleep, and making healthy choices about drugs and alcohol. If you work in a school library, make sure to let the guidance counselors know you have this book available. It includes fifteen downloadable guided meditations that you can use for teen/young adult programming.

The Mindful Twenty-Something: Life Skills to Handle Stress . . . & Everything Else by Holly B. Rogers.
Oakland, CA: New Harbinger, 2016. ISBN-1-62625-489-3; Paperback; US$16.95.

Here's a great book to target that elusive patron demographic: the emerging adult. The author is a counselor and mindfulness teacher at Duke University and creator of the evidence-based Koru Mindfulness program designed to teach stress reduction to college-age adults (there's even an app for it!).[7] Her focus on this age bracket really shows through the light, conversational style of the book that is informative but never patronizing. The book is full of helpful, easy-to-follow advice and thought experiments young adults can use to test out mindfulness practices for themselves. Some of these exercises could be used during a Stress Less for Teens program (see page 96) at your library.

SUGGESTIONS FOR PROFESSIONAL DEVELOPMENT COLLECTION

Teen Yoga for Yoga Therapists: A Guide to Development, Mental Health and Working with Common Teen Issues by Charlotta Martinus.
Philadelphia: Singing Dragon, 2018. ISBN 978-1848193994; Paperback; US$32.95/Can$45.95.

While appearing to be designed specifically for yoga therapists working closely with teens in crisis, this comprehensive guide offers wisdom to anyone teaching yoga to adolescents, or teaching yoga in general. The first part of the book details the brain chemistry of teens, what's going on in their bodies, how they react to society, and how yoga can help. The next section gets into typical teen issues such as eating disorders, anxiety, depression, sleep problems, bullying, exam stress, and troubled relationships. The third section concludes with ways to support teens in order to lead them to greater well-being and success. It also includes helpful charts and infographics. An excellent resource for those wanting to best serve this age group.

Yoga Exercises for Teens: Developing a Calmer Mind and a Stronger Body by Helen Purperhart.
Alameda, CA: Hunter House Publishers, 2009. ISBN 978-0897935036; Paperback; US$14.95/Can$19.50.

Purperhart's straightforward book is aimed at adolescents but has a special section called "Information for the Teacher" with an iconography, practical tips,

(*continued*)

and research into teens' actual experience of the practice, including direct quotes from students. This is very useful for library professionals who would like to start offering teen yoga programs. The rest of the book is dedicated to *Asanas* (some illustrated, some not), in series and sequences, as well as partner poses, meditations, and visualizations. While the book is marketed to teens, I think some students will have a hard time engaging in her non-visual directives for many of the exercises, as well as some of the sensible (but eye-roll-worthy) pose names, like "Crotch Stretch" and "Thumb" (a pose where you literally give the thumbs-up sign while smiling and saying, "I value myself"). Self-conscious teens may find all this a bit much. I'd relegate its usefulness for professional development, which is unfortunate because there aren't a lot of yoga books written for teens and young adults.[8]

Key Points

- When offering yoga and meditation to teens and young adults, remember they are generally self-conscious, under pressure to perform well (and look cool), and experiencing massive changes to their brain chemistry and hormones. The average prefrontal cortex doesn't finish developing the skills for emotional self-regulation until the early thirties, so cut teens some slack.[9] They might *want* to make good choices, they just might not always have the ability yet.
- This age group spans a wide range of development. Program models can be adapted to meet the needs of younger teens, late teens, and those in their twenties.
- Incorporating multimodal literacy components into these programs is easy when there are so many elements present in each program model: movement, writing opportunities, storytelling and sharing, reading, and music. This benefits different learning styles.
- Collection development of yoga and meditation materials for teens and young adults is important, and there are currently limited resources on the market for both the general public and for professional use. As we continue to promote yoga and meditation to this age demographic, we can hope that more resources will become available.

Notes

1. Deane Juhan, *Job's Body: A Handbook for Bodywork* (Barrytown, NY: Station Hill, 2003).

2. Bernadette Fulweiler and Rita Marie John, "Mind & Body Practices in the Treatment of Adolescent Anxiety," *Nurse Practitioner* 43, no. 8 (August 2018): 36–43.

3. See www.jenncarson.com.

4. Gina M. Biegel, *Be Mindful & Stress Less* (Boulder, CO: Shambhala, 2018).

5. Stressed Teens, "Stress and Mindfulness," Stressed Teens: Resources, accessed November 16, 2018, https://www.stressedteens.com/.

6. A previous version of this review is found at www.yogainthelibrary.com.

7. Centre for Koru Mindfulness, "About," Centre for Koru Mindfulness, accessed November 10, 2018, https://korumindfulness.org/.

8. A previous version of this review is found at www.yogainthelibrary.com.

9. William Stixrud and Ned Johnson, *The Self-Driven Child: The Science and Sense of Giving Your Kids More Control over Their Lives* (New York: Viking, 2018).

Yoga and Meditation for Adults and Seniors

Yoga and Meditation Programs for Adults and Seniors

THE MAJORITY OF yoga and meditation classes I teach in the library are geared toward adults, and about 60 percent of those who attend on any given day are over age fifty, both male and female. Some are even in their seventies and eighties. While most are in excellent physical condition, I do get people with hip replacements, shoulder replacements, scoliosis, arthritis, depression, bad knees, lower back pain, and some with autoimmune disorders or recovering from cancer. But this is true of any class, with any age demographic, because I also teach yoga at the Brazilian Jiu Jitsu gym where I train, and the guys there have bad shoulders, persistent soft tissue injuries, mental health issues, broken bones, and messed up necks, even though they exercise regularly and are fairly young and fit. The most important thing to keep in mind is that every *body* is different and to offer as many modifications as possible for each pose to help each student feel successful. When teaching meditation, start small, and remember that old habits are hard to break and sometimes the older we get the more difficult it can be to incorporate new habits into our routines. Celebrate small victories. The road to mindfulness is always rewarding, no matter when or how we start walking it.

◎ Program Models for Adults and Seniors

The following pages will offer a variety of programs designed to serve this age demographic at your library. While none of these programs are specifically designed "for seniors," they could certainly be marketed that way if you were trying to single out that segment of your population. Personally, I rarely think in such divisive terms. Many of my older students have as much energy and drive as my younger ones. Gentle Yoga (see below) is designed to introduce yoga at your library to beginners or those who would like a calm, restorative approach to the practice. Introduction to Meditation (page 109) provides a short but thorough immersion in multiple mindfulness practices that contribute to well-being. Yoga Minds Book Club (page 113) is a provocative program to get people thinking about mindfulness using mainstream books as a jumping-off point. It has discussion prompts for four popular titles to get you started, with suggestions for more.

◎ Program Model: Gentle Yoga

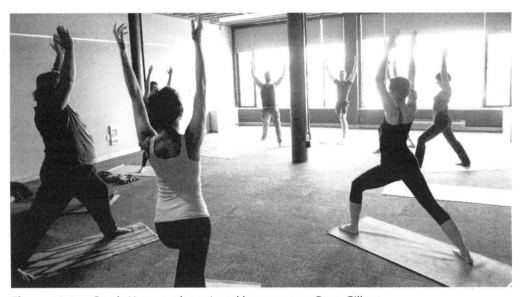

Figure 10.1. Gentle Yoga can be enjoyed by everyone. *Drew Gilbert*

This program is suitable for all levels and can be modified for most abilities. Can be done indoors or in the park, so you can practice in any weather!

Advance Planning

Step 1. Pick a time and date for the program. If you are aiming to attract seniors, daytime is best. For most working adults, evenings, weekends, and noon hours are more accessible. But keep in mind that many people also work shift work or from home and may be able to attend classes during a weekday. Plan for the session to be one hour.

Step 2. Book the room you'll be using.

Step 3. Decide whether the class is going to be a one-hit wonder or a regular weekly or monthly event. You could try it and if you get a good response, book more sessions. You'll also need to decide whether it is going to be a drop-in or pre-register session. At my library I offer it every Wednesday at noon, year-round.

Step 4. Secure a yoga teacher if you aren't planning on teaching the class yourself. Local yoga studios may have teachers, or teachers-in-training, willing to volunteer their time. Secure funding to pay for the teacher if you can't find a volunteer.

Step 5. Gather all necessary resources (see "Materials Required" section below).

Step 6. Prepare your paperwork (liability waivers, sign-up sheets, photo release forms, etc.). You may also want to print off copies of the routine to hand out so students can practice at home, or provide them with a digital link.[1] Consider administering a short evaluation form at the end to gauge how your audience felt.

Step 7. Familiarize yourself with the yoga sequence (see infographic on pages 106–108) or discuss with your hired instructor what they will be teaching.

Step 8. Advertise the event. Make a poster and put it up at places like the post office, town hall, medical clinics, and so forth. Add it to your online and print event calendar. Make a Facebook event to share. Call in to the radio and make a public service announcement—free yoga for seniors!

Step 9. Make a display of yoga-related material to refer patrons to after class.

Materials Required

- Mats, blocks, and straps for all participants (you may also want a few chairs handy for patrons with limited mobility in case you need to make modifications)
- Singing bowl or bell
- Liability waivers, photo release forms, evaluation forms, and other handouts
- Consent cards, if you plan to give hands-on adjustments

Budget Details

$0–$200+. This should be a relatively no-cost program if you already have all the mats and props you need. It's going to be significantly more expensive if you have to buy everything from scratch, but you could always ask patrons to bring their own mats, or apply for a grant. There is usually funding available for wellness or fitness programs for seniors. It may cost between $20–$100 to hire an instructor.

Day of Event

Step 1. Prepare the room by putting out all the mats and props.

Step 2. Welcome everyone as they arrive and have everyone complete a liability waiver/photo release (if you are taking pictures). Remind everyone to only do what feels good for their body and to not push beyond that.

Step 3. Follow along with the poses and instructions on the infographic (see pages 106–108). If you need to offer modifications for those who need to use a chair, please see the Chair Yoga program model in chapter 11 on pages 143–144.

Step 4. Bring everyone out of the final *Savasana* by ringing the bell/singing bowl.

Step 5. Thank everyone for coming. Give out evaluation forms to participants to encourage them to share how they felt during the practice anonymously and to offer any advice for how to best suit their needs during the next session.

Step 6. Refer patrons to your display of yoga-related materials in the library.

Step 7. Clean up and record your stats!

Gentle Yoga

A sweet and simple class designed for the absolute beginner, with more challenging options for those who want to take it to the next level.

1. Belly Breathing
Lie on the back with a bean bag placed on the belly. The feet roll out to the sides and the palms turn up to face the ceiling. Take a deep breath and feel the bean bag lift toward the ceiling, on the exhale feel the bean bag lower toward the spine. Repeat 5 times.

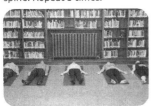

2. Ankle Rotations
Point and flex the toes 5 times. Turn the feet clockwise for 5 rotations. Turn counterclockwise for 5 rotations.

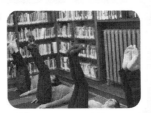

3. Knee Rotations
Holding on to the knees, circle the knees outward for 5 rotations. Circle inward for 5 rotations.

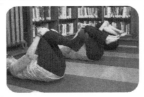

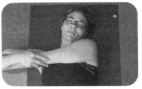

4. Shoulder Stretch
From lying on the back with legs out long, reach arms toward the ceiling and grasp opposite elbows. Gently rock arms to the left, moving across the chest. Gently rock arms to the right. Continue rocking back and forth across the body. Add head movement, following arms, if that feels good for the neck. Repeat 20 times.

5. Hip Rotations
Lift the right leg and point the toes toward the ceiling. Rotate the entire leg clockwise like tracing a golf ball with the big toe. After a few rotations, increase the size to a softball. Then a basketball. Then a beach ball. Then a hula hoop. Repeat rotations in same increments going counterclockwise. Lower the right leg and take a break. Then repeat entire sequence with the left leg.

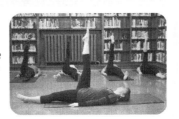

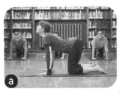

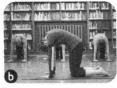

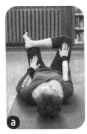

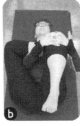

6. Figure 4
(a) Place the feet flat on the floor with the knees pointing toward the ceiling. Cross the right ankle over the left knee and use the right hand to push gently on the right knee. Point the right toes toward the ceiling. (b) Reach the right hand between the thighs and grasp either behind the left knee or on top of the left knee with both hands. Lower both knees toward the chest and take 5 breaths. Repeat entire sequence on the left side.

8. Cat/Cow Pose
(a) From a kneeling position, place both hands on the floor, shoulder-width apart. Press through the palms. Inhale and look toward the ceiling. (b) Exhale and arch the back upward, tucking the chin. Repeat both poses 9 more times.

7. Piriformis Stretch
(a) Place feet flat on the floor and cross the right knee over the left. Lower both knees toward the chest and hold the knees with both hands. Hold for 5 breaths. (b) For a deeper stretch: reach up, hold the feet, and gently pull them toward the floor.

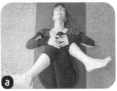

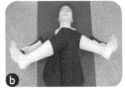

Program design by Jenn Carson   Photography by Ebony Scott   Layout by Samuel Holmes

Figure 10.2.

Gentle Yoga

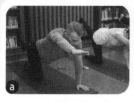
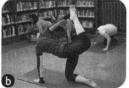

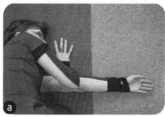

9. Kneeling Balance

(a) From a kneeling position lift the right hand and reach forward while lifting the left leg and reaching backward, like being pulled in two directions. (b) Reach back and gently grasp the left foot with the right hand. Take 5 breaths. If this is too difficult, repeat (a). (c) Bend the right arm to a 90° angle and lift beside the body. Bend the left leg the same way and lift, like peeing on a fire hydrant! (d) Straighten the right arm and straighten the left leg. Hold 5 breaths. Repeat the entire sequence, switching sides.

10. Kneeling Shoulder Stretches

(a) From a kneeling position, reach the left arm under the body, coming down onto the left shoulder. The left ear should be on the ground (or close). Keep the right hand planted on the floor. Take 5 breaths. (b) For a more advanced version, lift the right arm in the air. Repeat entire sequence on the right shoulder.

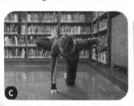
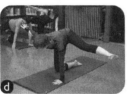

11. Down Dog

From a kneeling position, curl the toes under and place the hands shoulder-width apart. Push into palms and lift the hips in the air, lowering heels toward the floor, creating an inverted V shape. Line the ears up with the elbows. Lift the pinkie toes to externally rotate the thighs. Take 5 deep breaths. Step feet between the hands and come into standing.

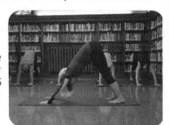

12. Six Essential Movements of the Spine

(a) From a standing position, reach arms overhead and clasp hands, releasing index fingers towards the ceiling. Inhale. Exhale and lean to the right. Inhale and come back up. Exhale and lean to the left. Inhale back up. Exhale and twist to the right. Inhale back to center. Exhale and twist to the left. (c) Inhale and come back to center. Exhale and look up to the ceiling. Inhale back to center. (d) Exhale and lower the arms to the floor. Slowly, moving one vertebrae at a time, roll the spine back to a standing position.

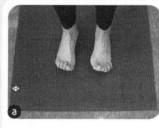

13. Mountain Pose

(a) From standing lift the toes and lower them slowly, feeling the floor solid underfoot. (b) Lift heart toward the ceiling. Relax the shoulders. Relax the jaw. Keep the pelvis neutral. Take 5 breaths.

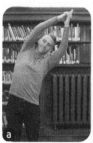
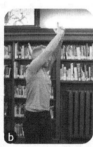
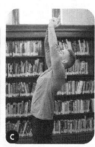
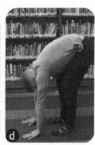

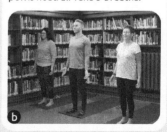

www.jenncarson.com
www.yogainthelibrary.com
www.physicalliteracyinthelibrary.com

Figure 10.3.

Gentle Yoga

Jenn Carson is a physical literacy expert, yoga instructor, librarian, and author of *Get Your Community Moving: Physical Literacy Programs For All Ages.*

14. Shoulder Rotations
(a) From a standing position, raise the arms out to the sides, at shoulder height, fingertips pointing to the ceiling. Rotate the arms in small circles going clockwise (backward). Gradually make the circles larger and larger. Repeat until the arms fatigue. Rest. (b) Repeat, this time with fingertips pointing to the floor and the arms rotating in small circles going counterclockwise (forward).

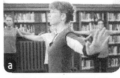
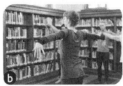

15. Tree Pose
Turn the right foot to a 90° angle. Lift the right foot to the left ankle. Option to lift to the calf or thigh instead (as shown). Bring the hands in prayer pose to the center of chest or raise arms overhead. Take 5 breaths. Lower the foot and repeat on the left side.

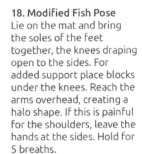

16. Chair Pose
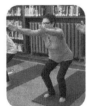
From a standing position with feet hip-width apart, bend the knees and drop the hips toward the ankles. Reach the arms forward, palms facing in. For more of a challenge, reach the arms overheard and sit lower, pressing through the heels.

17. Moving Bridge Pose
(a) Lie on the back with the feet planted on the floor and the knees pointing toward the ceiling. (b) Inhale and lift the hips upward and raise the arms overhead. Exhale and lower the hips and arms. Repeat 4 more times.

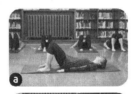
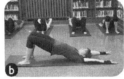

18. Modified Fish Pose
Lie on the mat and bring the soles of the feet together, the knees draping open to the sides. For added support place blocks under the knees. Reach the arms overhead, creating a halo shape. If this is painful for the shoulders, leave the hands at the sides. Hold for 5 breaths.

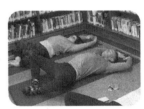

19. Bound Forward Bend
(a) From an easy sitting position (or Lotus or Half-Lotus) reach behind the back and hold the opposite elbows or wrists. Inhale and look toward the ceiling. Exhale and fold torso over the knees. (b) For more of a challenge, lower the head to the mat or a block. Hold for 5 breaths.

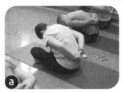
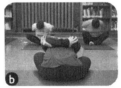

22. *Savasana*
Lie on the mat with a bean bag on the belly. Roll the feet to the sides and the palms toward the ceiling. Close the eyes and continue with Belly Breathing for at least 5 minutes.

20. Meditation Pose
Sitting in an easy crossed-leg position (or Lotus or Half-Lotus) place the back of wrists on the fronts of knees. Tuck the index finger under thumb. Straighten the other three fingers toward the floor. Tuck the chin and close the eyes, or gaze softly ahead. Hold for 10 breaths.

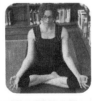

21. Uplifting Pose
Cross the ankles. (a) Place the hands on blocks or on the mat next to hips. Lift the knees and lift the bottom off the mat. (b) Option to lift hands and hover. Hold for 5 breaths. Lower to the ground.

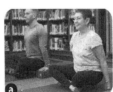
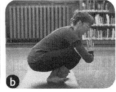

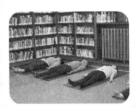

Figure 10.4.

Advice

- Remember it is a class designed for beginners, but don't be afraid to offer modifications to those who may wish to take the pose deeper. You can explain they are optional. Likewise, offer plenty of alternatives for those who have injuries or issues. For example, for those who can't do the Figure 4 Pose on the ground, they may be more comfortable doing it with their feet pressing against a wall. For those who have a hard time doing Piriformis Stretch, offer them Shoelace Pose from a seated position.
- Remind everyone that they can always come into Child's Pose or Easy Pose if they need a rest.
- People may talk during class, especially if they are nervous. Try not to make too much of it.
- Don't forget to offer consent cards or ask people to let you know if they don't want to be touched during hands-on assists (if you are offering).

⑥ Program Model: Introduction to Meditation

This simple program offers a low-key introduction to meditation for the curious. It can be held as a one-time event, or offered on a weekly or monthly basis. It can also easily be adapted as an outreach program, or expanded as a half-day workshop (see "Advice" section for more details).

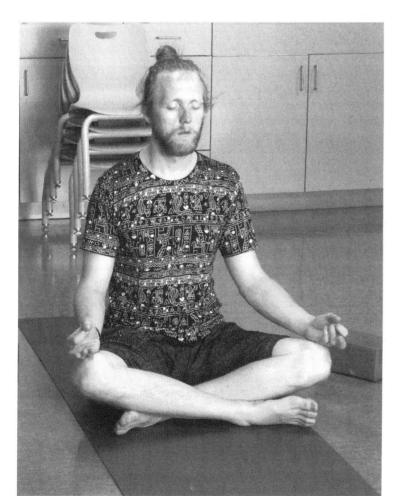

Figure 10.5. Meditation for beginners.
Brendan Helmuth

Advance Planning

Step 1. Decide whether you feel comfortable leading the program yourself (or have a staff member with meditation experience who could step in) and if not, seek out a meditation instructor in your community. Good places to look are local meditation centers, yoga studios, or university campuses. If you don't meditate regularly, don't teach meditation.[2]

Step 2. Once you secure a teacher, or have read over the materials several times yourself, pick a time and date and book a room (a quiet one!). If you know the library is super loud after school, for example, that might not be the best time. Evenings or weekends are best if you want to target working professionals; during the day works well for seniors, or those who work shift work. Lunchtime is also a good option to catch people on their break from work. A beginner session like this should last no more than thirty to forty-five minutes.

Step 3. Decide whether this will be a one-off program or an ongoing weekly or monthly event. You could try it once and if the people who show up are enthusiastic, offer it more regularly. I wouldn't recommend having more than five to ten people at a time, so you may want to make it registration only.

Step 4. Gather all the materials listed below.

Step 5. Advertise your event. Make a print poster. Make a Facebook event. Put it on your website and event calendar. Tweet about it. Make sure to mention it at the circulation desk to anyone checking out meditation-related books.

Step 6. Do the paperwork. Make a sign-up sheet if you require registration. Prepare photo release waivers if you plan on taking photos/videos of the event (though most people won't want to have their picture taken or be recorded while meditating, so I advise against this). Short evaluation forms are helpful and recommended.

Materials Required

- Singing bowl or bell
- Meditation cushions or chairs
- A display of meditation books (don't forget audiobooks and CDs too!)
- A room large enough to walk in a circle with five to ten people, or access to an outdoor space where you can walk relatively undisturbed, such as a park with a path, an empty ball field, or a large lawn
- A clock, phone, or watch for timing sessions

Budget Details

$0. The program shouldn't cost anything, unless you want to buy some fancy meditation cushions. You can easily use existing library chairs, and if you don't have a singing bowl or bell, use the timer and bell on your phone. Any meditation instructor I've ever recruited has never charged.

Day of Event

Step 1. Set up the room (see the "Advice" section for suggestions).

Step 2. Greet students as they arrive. Introduce yourself (and the instructor if you've recruited one) and thank everyone for joining. Have them complete any required paperwork. Depending on the size of the group you may wish to have everyone go around and introduce themselves (works well with eight or fewer people), or jump right in.

Step 3. Explain what mindfulness is: the ability to recognize what is going on in the mind, body, and surroundings, without getting caught up by it. We use the practice of *noticing* the thought, sensation, or environmental input, and then we look at it with a sort of friendly curiosity, without judgment. If we do have a reaction, like irritation, we watch that too. Like, "Hmm, look at that, I'm thinking about lunch. I'm hungry. And a little impatient because I want to eat now." We can even use this insight to have more compassion for our family, friends, and colleagues, or even strangers. Such as, "Hmm, Bob's a little cranky in this meeting, and it's almost noon. I wonder if he's hungry too." We learn to not internalize other people's behavior so much and realize that often how people react has very little to do with us. When we open in this way, we are both kinder to others and kinder to ourselves, because we realize the only person's behavior we really have any control over is our own. So change must start from within. We also lower our expectations. We cannot be happy all the time. Everything doesn't always work out the way we want it to. But, as Thich Nhat Hanh says, when we have a toothache we really appreciate the moments in our lives when we didn't have toothaches.[3] The trick is to remember these non-toothache moments when they are happening. How lucky we are to not have toothaches right now! When we stop wishing to change reality and instead just sit with "what is," we can begin to appreciate the ebb and flow of life and how the only constant is change. Of course, we forget. Because we are human. This is why we practice.

Step 4. Lead your students through a guided meditation practice. Choose one from your own tradition, read one from a book (see "Suggestions for Circulating Collection" textbox on page 120 for ideas), or use the one I've provided here. If you are using meditation cushions instead of chairs, adapt the language accordingly. Set the timer for five minutes.

GUIDED CHAIR MEDITATION FOR BEGINNERS

Come to sitting on the edge of your seat with your feet planted firmly on the floor. Have your hands resting in your lap in a way that is most comfortable for you. Close your eyes or gaze softly ahead, not focusing on anything. Draw your attention to the soles of the feet. Feel them heavy on the ground. Feel the weight of your hands in your lap. Relax your jaw and shoulders, allowing the tension to melt down toward the floor. Sit up comfortably, keeping your spine as straight as possible without strain. Notice your breath moving your belly in and out. Draw the attention to the nostrils now. As you inhale, notice the cool air from the room rushing over your nostrils. As you exhale, notice the warm air rushing out. Notice the pause between the inhale and the exhale. On the next inhale say to yourself, inside your head: "One." On the exhale, say, "Two." On the next inhale say, "Three." Continue counting each inhale and exhale until you get to ten, and then start all over again. If your mind wanders off into thought, just start all over again at "One." Continue this way until we ring the bell and end the session.

Step 5. Open the floor to discussion if people would like to share their experience while meditating. Some questions to prompt the sharing could include:

- That was five minutes; did it feel that long?
- Did you find it easy to stay on track with the counting, or did you have to start over and over again?
- Did you feel fidgety, or was it comfortable to sit still?
- Were you distracted by anything in the environment? If so, what did you do to bring your attention back to the breath?

Step 6. Have everyone come to standing and do a little stretch. Then have everyone line up single file and move to an open area (indoors or outdoors) where you can form a circle or walking line. Demonstrate how to do a walking meditation: very slowly, noticing each point of contact the foot makes with the ground, hands clasped behind the back or draping gently at the sides, gaze to the ground so as to minimize distractions, focusing on the breath and the body mechanics of each movement. Have everyone practice walking meditation for five minutes. Ring the bell to bring them out of it and have them return to their seats.

Step 7. Open the floor to discussion. This time they can compare the seated meditation to the walking meditation. Ask them to share any observations they had about the practice.

Step 8. Repeat steps 4 through 7 as many times as your session length allows, perhaps growing longer in duration with each repetition. For example, the second round could be for seven minutes, the third for ten, and so forth. You could ask students during the discussion if it felt any longer this time (don't tell them ahead of time you were making it longer).

Step 9. After your last meditation, bring everyone back to their chairs. Explain that this is the end of the session and see if they have any additional questions. Ask them if they are willing to commit to meditating for five minutes every day for a week and see if it makes a difference. Recommend some books for them to take home to encourage them in their practice (see "Suggestions for Circulating Collection" textbox on page 120) for suggestions for your display. Let them know of any upcoming mindfulness programs at the library or in the community. Hand out the evaluation forms, if using. Thank your facilitator, if you didn't lead the program yourself.

Step 10. Clean up and record your stats. Are you feeling any calmer from all that meditation? If not, take a few minutes for yourself before heading back to your desk or your next task.

Advice

- Set up the room with a row or two of chairs or cushions to accommodate the number of students who have registered. A circle can be too intimidating; everyone may feel that they are being looked at while they are meditating. Or they may find it too tempting to look at each other, which can be distracting to a beginner. It is best to have minimal distractions and a bland background. In Zen practice it is actually tradition to face a blank wall. If you have enough wall space you could try that, though for some patrons it may trigger memories from childhood of being punished.

- A great way to target busy urban professionals or students at academic libraries is to offer a thirty-minute lunch 'n' learn. They can bring their own bagged lunch (or if you have the budget, you can provide food) and they can eat while you run through the first few steps, explaining mindfulness. Then they can practice chewing mindfully, and once they are finished eating you can do a five-minute seated meditation and five-minute walking meditation. This short format allows them plenty of time to get back to class or the office and is a great way to attract people who may be too skeptical or busy to try a longer session.
- If you have the space in your programming schedule, think you would have the audience, and have the stamina and experience to teach it, I recommend expanding this program to a half- or full-day workshop. When I give the extended version of the program, I offer seated and walking meditation indoors, as well as a longer walk on a nearby nature trail (with the option to wear "silence" stickers for those who wish to be quiet; others may wish to engage in mindful conversation). We also practice eating our lunches mindfully in silence. And I give them all a copy of *Making Space: Creating a Home Meditation Practice* by Thich Nhat Hanh, along with leading a discussion about replicating our "retreat" atmosphere at home.

⊚ Program Model: Yoga Minds Book Club

A great way to get people interested in yoga and meditation who aren't ready to dive right into the practice is by having a book club on the topic. When you combine experienced practitioners with people who are learning about yoga and mindfulness for the first time, you could get lots of stimulating discussions! It's best to choose books that are easily relatable, are told in the first person, and read more like a story than a textbook. Save the explorations of Patanjali's *Yoga Sutras* or the Buddha's *Four Noble Truths* for your personal practice; what we want to use here are books that will draw in the general public and whet their appetite (no instruction manuals!). Think: celebrity forays into meditation, or funny memoirs of wine-chugging yoginis Down-Dogging their way to enlightenment. Here's a selection of four books to get you started, complete with ten discussion prompts each.

Advance Planning

Step 1. Gather the books listed in the "Materials Required" section and read them. Then read over the discussion prompts listed in the "Day of Event" section. Add your own prompts, as desired. Or choose different books. There are many more suggestions on page 120.

Step 2. Make sure you have enough copies of the books available in your library system as you think you might need. Order and add more copies, as required (and funding is available). Don't forget about alternative formats such as e-books, audiobooks, Playaways, braille books, and large print. Put a group hold on the titles for your book club (as permitted by your library's policies).

Step 3. Choose a date and time for the book club. Evenings are a good choice to get the most diverse audience. Will you meet monthly? Every two months? Will this be an ongoing event (hopefully never running out of books as more and more get published each year!)? Or will it be for a set time period (six months or six sessions, for example). Plan far enough in advance that people actually have time to read the book.

Step 4. Book the room needed for the program, preferably a place with comfy chairs or couches.

Step 5. Make sure you make up a schedule in advance of which books you are reading each month (or however often you are holding the book club) that you can share when you advertise the event and people sign up (if you are requiring registration). That way people can get a head start on reading. If you are making the book club registration only, make a sign-up sheet.

Step 6. Advertise the event. Make a poster. Give a copy to local yoga studios and meditation centers. Share on social media. Put it on your print and digital calendars. Share in your yoga and mindfulness programs. Tell anyone who checks out a book that is of related subject matter. Recruit your yoga friends. Bribe your mom. Tell anyone who isn't even interested in the topic but loves to read and talk about books to come; it will help generate discussion. If you have a room full of like-minded readers it is much less lively. A little controversy is a good thing.

Materials Required

- *10% Happier: How I Tamed the Voice in My Head, Reduced Stress without Losing My Edge, and Found Self-Help That Actually Works—A True Story* by Dan Harris
- *Poser: My Life in Twenty-Three Yoga Poses* by Claire Dederer
- *Single White Monk: Tales of Death, Failure, and Bad Sex (Although Not Necessarily in That Order)* by Shozan Jack Haubner
- *Yoga Bitch: One Woman's Quest to Conquer Skepticism, Cynicism, and Cigarettes on the Path to Enlightenment* by Suzanne Morrison

Budget Details

$0–$100+. If you already have all the books in your library system and enough available copies, this program is not going to cost you a penny. If you have to start buying copies of the books, it could get pricey.

Day of Event

Step 1. Welcome everyone to the group and do an icebreaker activity to help everyone get to know each other. Here's an example: have each person say their name and demonstrate a yoga pose they know or just made up.

Step 2. Start the session by going over the book of choice with a quick synopsis. I'm not sure the stats on how many people actually finish the book before attending a book club meeting in general, but I bet they are surprisingly low. This gives the slackers a chance to catch up without shame.

Step 3. Go through your discussion prompts. Don't be surprised if you don't get through all ten. People may have lots of opinions about these books. This is good! Here are the discussion questions, publishing information, and a short description of each book:

10% Happier: How I Tamed the Voice in My Head, Reduced Stress without Losing My Edge, and Found Self-Help That Actually Works—A True Story by Dan Harris.
New York: HarperCollins, 2014. ISBN 978-0-06-226543-2; Paperback; US$15.99/ Can$21.00.

Famous newscaster Dan Harris has a rude awakening when he succumbs to a panic attack on-screen for the first time. No stranger to pushing through obstacles, for years this war correspondent hid his anxiety, drug use, and undiagnosed depression from everyone he loved and worked for, even while in the literal trenches. In the hypercompetitive world of news reporting, Harris is terrified to show an iota of weakness, lest he lose his job—or worse, his sanity—until his body and mind do it for him, and he has to start figuring out a better way to live. Part memoir, part exposé of the wellness world's underbelly, and part love letter to the practice that finally saved him: meditation. Your Yoga Minds Book Club readers will enjoy Harris's biting self-deprecation and firsthand accounts of famous spiritual leaders like Eckhart Tolle and Deepak Chopra, who may not be as perfect as they seem on TV.

Book Club Questions (*warning: spoilers!*):

1. What was your interpretation of Harris's "war is a drug" approach to being a war correspondent, and his subsequent spiral into coke addiction when he got home? What do you think made him want to put himself in the line of fire in the first place?

2. How do you feel about the ongoing empathy Harris shows for Ted Haggard and his wife?

3. Harris describes Eckhart Tolle as "the type of person who, if you met him at a cocktail party, you would either ignore or avoid." Have you read any of Tolle's books or listened to his talks? What do you think of Harris's interpretation of him and his focus on "now"?

4. There is an ongoing refrain in the book that Harris comes back to over and over again: *Something minor but negative happens* (going bald shows up a lot) = *unemployment = Harris ends up in a flophouse in Duluth.* This sort of thinking is called "catastrophizing" by psychologists. Even though it might seem ridiculous from the outside, we all engage in it (some of us much more than others!). What's something you catastrophize about? How does Harris's meditation practice help him with this?

5. On page 104, Harris says that according to the Buddha, there are three habitual responses to the human experience: we want the experience, we don't want the experience, or we zone out. He uses these examples: "Cookies: I want. Mosquitos: I reject. The safety instructions the flight attendants read aloud on an airplane: I zone out." Mindfulness, he says, is the fourth option. We sit with what is. We observe the experience without desire or rejection, and we don't zone out either. By this point in the book, Harris is pretty sure this is impossible. What do you think?

6. At the end of Harris's meditation retreat, Goldstein urges his audience to run their thoughts through the filter of "Is this useful?" Have you ever noticed yourself ruminating about something, running it over and over in your mind? Even if it isn't upsetting, something as benign as mulling over your to-do list can be taken to excess. What would it feel like to free up your mental capacity if you only concentrated on "useful" thoughts and let the other ones go? How do you define a "useful" thought from an "un-useful" one?

7. Janice Marturano tells Harris to only do one thing at a time. When eating to pay attention only to eating. When talking on the phone to only do that. How would this one small change affect your entire day? Could you do it? Could you do it for even ten minutes?

8. Sharon Salzberg advises Harris, who is worried about being overlooked at work, that "often it's not the unknown that scares us, it's that we think we know what's going to happen—and that it is going to be bad. But the truth is, we really don't know." What's an example from the book, or from your own life, where you (or Harris) assumed the worst but it didn't happen?

9. At the end of the book Harris asks, "What matters most?" How has his approach to life radically changed from the beginning of the book to the end?

10. Do you meditate? If yes, how did reading it affect your practice? If not, did the book make you want to start?

Poser: My Life in Twenty-Three Yoga Poses by Claire Dederer.
New York: Picador, 2011. ISBN 978-1-250-00233-4; Paperback; US$17.00/Can$19.00.

In this best-selling mom-oir, journalist Claire Dederer meditates on what it means to be *good*: a good mother, a good wife, a good friend, a good citizen, a good sister, and a good daughter. She does it all through the lens of her increasingly all-consuming new hobby: yoga. While the book is formally structured around her exploration of these ideals from the vantage point of various yoga poses, the real arc of the narrative is how Dederer uses yoga and the insight gained from its practice to deal with her husband's depression, the vulgarity of her envy and judgment toward her friends, her own self-criticism, her body's limitations, and her increasing anger at her parents' refusal to get a divorce, even though her mother has been living with another (younger) man for a couple of decades. If this isn't enough fodder for the emotional-anguish fire, Dederer also hints at a childhood spiced with the kind of parental self-absorption (and subsequent drug/alcohol use) that leads to her having an (inebriated) family friend crawl into her sleeping bag in the middle of the night and proceed to do something alarming, the details of which are vague. Your book club members' impressions of Dederer's unvarnished opinions, and her turning toward yoga as a sort of salve and possible redemption from the tedium of her life, should make for interesting conversation indeed!

Book Club Questions (*warning: spoilers!*):

1. Early in chapter 2, Dederer says the following: "Maybe I was the only one who, grinding steamed organic carrots in the baby-food mill, felt as if turning the mill's little handle was keeping something awful from happening. . . . Having recently become a mother, I was surprised by the level of dread that filled me at almost all times. There was occasional pleasure, but it often consisted of the cessation of dread." Have any of you, once becoming parents, also experienced this feeling? How did it affect your day-to-day life and decisions?

2. Dederer describes the West-Coast-liberal-in-the-nineties/turn-of-the-century experience as being one of striving for a sort of moral good that surpassed the pedestrian, perhaps more superficial, "perfectionism" of their predecessors, and taking it to a new level of social paranoia. One where it isn't enough to appear to be good (by shopping at Whole Foods instead of IGA), but to actually scrub yourself clean of anything deemed as harmful by your peers (which is why you must walk to Whole Foods, while schlepping your reusable, sustainable-fabric bags, and not purchase anything with an iota of excessive packaging and preferably no packaging at all). Have you ever felt this requirement to take "goodness" to the level where you felt that every action must be unquestionably beyond reproach? Do you know anyone who does?

3. What was your opinion of Dederer's friend Lucy and her actions in the story? Did you find this character relatable?

4. What did you think of the dynamic between Dederer and her husband? Their tag-team approach to attending parties? Their sharing of email accounts and professions? Their mutual avoidance of addressing his depression and her anxiety?

5. How do you think Dederer's increasing interest in yoga affected her relationship to her husband? Her friends? Herself?

6. Do you think there was any correlation between Dederer's need to be an exemplary mother and her own mother's behavior when she was a child? How about her mother's behavior now? What did you think about the scene at the party when her mother insists on moving the dining room table to make the atmosphere just right and Dederer's reaction to it?

7. What did you think about the family's move to Colorado and its timing? Should they have stayed in Colorado longer?

8. For most of the book Dederer finds herself confronted with lithe, impossibly beautiful, spandex-wearing teachers half her age, going through banal expressions of what it means to practice yoga. When Dederer starts attending Seidel's classes in a strip mall near the end of the book—and finds an unpretentious middle-aged woman in a frumpy T-shirt guiding her to just let the structure of her body do the work instead of always "muscling" into the pose—how does this affect the author's practice? What did you think of Seidel's reply to Dederer's question about what she was supposed to be "feeling" in the pose: "What are we supposed to be feeling? Who knows? We're working with the subtle body. It's gonna surprise us. We just have to get out of the way."

9. Near the end of the book, the author's teacher Seidel encourages her to accept her limitations, to think of yoga as a "counterweight" to the way she behaves in the rest of her life, using the example of enjoying having the feeling of open shoulders for the duration of class even if you know you will go back to hunching them the minute you leave. In what way is practicing yoga like other spiritual traditions where you pay penance, have confession, and go back out in the world trying to be a little better? How does this approach affect Dederer's obsessive need to be "good" at all times? By the end of the book can you feel her softening in her approach to anything? How did it affect your opinion of what a yoga practice should be?

10. At the end of the book Dederer moves home to the island where her life first fell apart. What maturation process do you think was required of her to achieve this homecoming? Have you ever revisited a place where something devastating happened to you?

Single White Monk: Tales of Death, Failure, and Bad Sex (Although Not Necessarily in That Order) by Shozan Jack Haubner.
Boulder, CO: Shambhala, 2017. ISBN 978-1-61180-363-1; Paperback; US$14.95/ Can$19.95.

Many of us have an idealized vision of what the life of a Buddhist monk must look like: long periods of peaceful contemplation, communal meals with fellow bald and saffron-robed companions, a life free from financial stresses and romantic complications . . . perhaps even enlightenment (whatever that is). Well, a Zen priest with the pen name of Shozan Jack Haubner is about to crumble that nice little fairy tale into soiled, scratchy toilet paper and throw it at your face while laughing maniacally.

Welcome to the trenches of spiritual warfare: they involve sex scandals, illness, death, drugs, prostitution, and copious amounts of self-loathing sprinkled with humor. This book is not for anyone who intends to keep the veil of Buddhist purity firmly in place. I guarantee your Yoga Minds participants will have strong feelings about this memoir, and they won't all be positive.

Book Club Questions (*warning: spoilers!*):

1. What sort of feelings came up when you read Haubner's account of his encounter at the massage parlor on his birthday? Did this chapter make him more relatable as a narrator, or less?

2. On page 36 Haubner says, "This is the First Noble Truth in Buddhism: everyone's broken. If you take these words seriously . . . then you know that our brokenness doesn't need fixing. It needs company. I used to think that being an adult meant being self-sufficient. These days I think it means realizing that the self is never sufficient. That's just not the way we're built." What do those words mean to you? What do you think it means to be an adult? Would we be happier if we could just accept and share our imperfections?

3. In chapter 7, Haubner becomes violently ill. He says, "Patience is key to your mental health when you are ill . . . for your life is now on hold." Has there ever been a time you've felt like that? What about when someone you love is sick? Do you think Haubner could be described as patient in this chapter?

4. While recovering from his illness, Haubner visits a Catholic priest and tells him he's on the verge of quitting the monastic life and asks if he ever gets tired of his religious career path. The priest replies that all of life is tiresome. He tells Haubner that every man has demons and that you can't fight them or fall under their spell, but must instead surrender to them. What do you think he meant by that?

5. After Haubner's "dark night of the soul" in his parents' garage he tells himself to "get it together" if not for himself, then for his mom. He then comes to the realization that during his three months recovering from his illness he'd forgotten the most basic principle of meditation: "Breathe into the place where you ache the most." The act of thinking, he discovers, or being attached to that thinking, is the real disease. Can you relate to this experience he shares? For those with experience meditating, how do you stay with the breath when you are in the most pain?

6. When Haubner's laptop gets stolen he's sitting in the police station obsessively checking his phone. He notices himself doing this but can't seem to stop. He concludes that perhaps meditation has "simply honed my awareness to the point where I can clearly see how imperfect I am but has in no way helped me to change this fact." Do you think it's better to be aware of your flaws—even if you feel helpless to do anything to change them—or to be blissfully ignorant of your neuroses and dysfunctional social conditioning?

7. Haubner introduces us to a monk named Daishin through his death. He discusses how Daishin never pretended to be anything other than he was, a deeply disturbed and unique individual, beloved by those closest to him. Do you know anyone like that? Someone who is fully themselves—warts and all? How do you feel when they are around?

8. As Daishin is dying, Haubner struggles to resist the urge to save him and to instead help him let go. This requires a massive letting go for both of them. Haubner

calls this a "surrender bender." Meanwhile, Daishin is still getting up and trying to walk around and reassuring his grieving guests they can still visit him in the hospital when hospice comes to collect him. Can we accept death joyfully? What does "letting go" mean to you?

9. During the sex scandal Haubner reports that Roshi only wrote one apology that never went public. The only lines Haubner remembers are, "I made too many mistakes. Trying to teach is already a mistake." Haubner writes an apology on behalf of the organization that did go public. Why do you think he felt compelled to become the voice of the *Sangha* (meditation community)?

10. Haubner argues with Lizzie on page 154 to the point of physical violence. He never explicitly says who hit who first. Does it matter? Later, he describes a scene of Lizzie being attacked by Roshi. Were you expecting there to be so much violence in a story about monks and nuns? What do you think it says about our culture and human nature that in a community lauded for its peacefulness so much aggression abounds?

Yoga Bitch: One Woman's Quest to Conquer Skepticism, Cynicism, and Cigarettes on the Path to Enlightenment by Suzanne Morrison.
New York: Three Rivers Press, 2011. ISBN 978-0307717443; Paperback; US$16.00/Can$21.00.

What happens when a wine-swilling, cigarette-loving, meat-eating, morally questionable twenty-five-year-old embarks on a two-month yoga teacher training retreat in Bali a few months before she is set to move to New York City with the love of her life? Everything. Suzanne Morrison lands in sweltering, buggy, stray-dog-infested Bali only to discover her fellow yogis drink their own pee, abstain from all sex (including self-love), and have very strong opinions about *Samtosha* (contentment). It is a coming-of-age tale for the Down Dog generation, filled with (repressed) lust, late night, high-calorie debauchery, disillusion with enlightenment, and some surprisingly tender plot twists.

Book Club Questions (*warning: spoilers!*):

1. What was your impression of Indra at the beginning of the book? How did it change by the end of the book?

2. What was your impression of Lou at the beginning of the book? How did it change by the end of the book?

3. Indra and Lou are based on real people; how do you think they reacted to being described by Morrison, her evolving feelings for them, and to the intimate details of their lives being exposed? Do you think Lou knew about Morrison's stealing at the studio?

4. Morrison said she never really used her yoga teacher training when she returned from Bali, even though she enjoyed teaching. Why do you think this is?

5. Were you surprised she went to New York? Why or why not?

6. What was your impression of Jessica? Do you think you would have liked having her for a roommate?

7. Would you try urine therapy? Why or why not?

8. How did you feel at the end of the book when Morrison and her friends indulged in brownies and alcohol after all their abstention? Did this make you like them more, or less?

9. There is an interesting underlying thread running through the book about our attachment to objects, especially those of sentimental value. What did you think of Jessica's purchasing of shoes for a wedding she was certain she would have someday with a man she hadn't even met yet? What about Morrison's coveting of the expensive purse? Would you have bought it? When have you felt like an object of desire just wouldn't stop taunting you? Do you think it is possible to relinquish our materialism? How much of it is culturally manifested and how much is naturally ingrained because of our need for survival?

10. What do you think was the biggest lesson Morrison learned in Bali? What did you learn from reading this book?

OTHER SUGGESTIONS FOR YOGA MINDS BOOK CLUB

- *The Dude and the Zen Master* by Jeff Bridges and Bernie Glassman
- *Eat Pray Love* by Elizabeth Gilbert
- *Hell-Bent: Obsession, Pain, and the Search for Something Like Transcendence in Competitive Yoga* by Benjamin Lorr
- *Holy Cow: An Indian Adventure* by Sarah Macdonald
- *The Power of Now: A Guide to Spiritual Enlightenment* by Eckhart Tolle
- *Siddhartha* by Hermann Hesse
- *Stretch: The Unlikely Making of a Yoga Dude* by Neal Pollack
- *The Tao of Pooh* by Benjamin Hoff
- *Wellmania: Extreme Misadventures in the Search for Wellness* by Brigid Delaney

Advice

- This is an excellent program to use for outreach. Consider hosting the book club at a local meditation or yoga studio, hospital, health center, prison, or adult education center.
- If your book club is going to be for a set number of sessions (say, four or six), consider offering a mini yoga class or meditation session at the closing party of the last session.
- This program also works well with teens and university students; however, some of the subject matter in the books may be a bit too mature for younger teens, so I would keep it age eighteen and up.

SUGGESTIONS FOR CIRCULATING COLLECTION

Bliss More: How to Succeed in Meditation without Really Trying by Light Watkins. New York: Ballantine Books, 2018. ISBN 978-0-399-18035-4; Hardcover; US$24.00/Can$32.00.

If you can help your patrons get past the title and cover of this book, with its puffy clouds and tampon-box color scheme, they would discover an accessible and easygoing manual on how to meditate for beginners. Despite seeming like a new-agey guide written by a caftan-wearing white woman, the author (yes, whose chosen name is Light) is actually a black dude from Alabama who used to be a fashion model and then took up teaching yoga and hosting consciousness-raising dinner parties. So, alongside dropping our stereotypical views of who a meditation teacher is, Watkins asks us to also drop our preconceived notions of how meditation is supposed to be done. He makes the analogy that you wouldn't expect a beginner jogger to train like an Olympic athlete, and so there is no reason to expect a beginner meditator to sit up in a lotus position for thirty-plus minutes clearing their mind. Instead he advocates for comfortable seating—wherever you happen to find yourself—permission to glance at the clock and wander into thought, and minimal time allotments for sittings. He calls his approach the E.A.S.Y. method, and it will surely appeal to those skeptical patrons who would like to try meditation, but don't see themselves shaving their heads and donning saffron-colored robes anytime soon.

Every Body Yoga: Let Go of Fear, Get on the Mat, Love Your Body by Jessamyn Stanley. New York: Workman, 2017. ISBN 978-0-7611-9311-1; Paperback; US$16.95/Can$24.95.

Jessamyn Stanley is a black, queer, overweight, body-positive, and very popular yoga teacher who will straight-talk you through how to begin a yoga practice. I do not recommend this book to anyone who is offended by swearing (lots and lots of swearing). But it answers some of those questions people might be too embarrassed to ask in your classes, such as "What if I fart during class?" or "What if I'm the fattest person in class and everyone stares at me?" (spoiler: her answer to both is pretty much, "Who cares?"). Stanley discusses her difficult childhood, issues with body image and addiction, and what led her to yoga in the first place. But this book is not to be taken as a biography, even if she does use her own struggles as a framework for the sequences. The sequences themselves are well explained, and actually doable, and the models are normal-looking people (for example: a balding, average-weight guy and a tattooed, hairy-arm-pitted, semi-shaved-head lady). Clothes are often wrinkled and riding up. No one looks like they just stepped off the cover of *Yoga Journal*. A certain demographic of your patrons is going to find a book like this incredibly refreshing, and I recommend having it around to display during classes or to hand out to nervous new students, regardless of their body weight.

The Joy of Yoga: Fifty Sequences for Your Home and Studio Practice by Emma Silverman. New York: Skyhorse, 2018. ISBN 978-1-5107-2393-1; Paperback; US$14.99/Can$22.99.

The beauty and effectiveness of this book is in its simplicity. There are no complicated, medical-jargon-laden explanations of the poses, just fifty easy-to-follow sequences with clear photographs of a model demonstrating the most typical expression of each pose. Each pose is named in English and Sanskrit, and while there are occasional modification suggestions in the sequence description, they are rare, so this book is best for the independent yogi looking for some straightforward sequences to practice or teach. The sequences are divided by subject (for example, "The Great Outdoors" or "Planes, Trains and Automobiles"). Here's some samples from various

(*continued*)

chapters: "Yoga for People Who Type Too Much," "Yoga for Menstruation," "Yoga Poses That Are Awkward to Do Naked," "Yoga for Anger Management," and "Yoga for Sensitive Wrists." An excellent addition to your circulating collection.

Making Space: Creating a Home Meditation Practice by Thich Nhat Hanh.
Berkeley, CA: Parallax Press, 2012. ISBN 978-1-937006-00-6; Paperback; US$9.95/Can$13.50.

This essential little book (only ninety-two tiny pages!) gets given out at every meditation retreat I teach (thanks to generous grants through my provincial government's wellness program). Nhat Hanh has created short, accessible chapters on a few different approaches to meditation, soothing mantras, and advice for how to set up your home and life to make it more peaceful by including mindful eating, a breathing space, and a calm sleeping space, and how to include family members in your quest for a more restful and aware existence. I especially enjoy "The Cake in the Refrigerator" exercise for restoring harmony in times of family discord. Besides adding to the circulating collection, this book makes a thoughtful gift for employees, volunteers, or library stakeholders involved in meditation or looking for ways to de-stress their lives.

Meditation for Fidgety Skeptics: A 10% Happier How-To Book by Dan Harris, Jeff Warren, and Carlye Adler.
New York: Spiegel & Grau, 2017. ISBN 978-0-399-58894-5; Hardcover; US$26.00/Can$35.00.

While at first it may seem like a cash grab for Harris to write a follow-up how-to manual to go with 2014's best-selling meditation memoir *10% Happier: How I Tamed the Voice in My Head, Reduced Stress without Losing My Edge, and Found Self-Help That Actually Works—A True Story* (see page 115 for a description), they are both such self-deprecating and wildly narcissistic books (traits also surprisingly embodied in one very funny man) it's worth having both on the shelf. Perhaps it will draw the attention of potential meditators that may respect Harris for his newscasting and not know about this other side of his life. These are the books Harris writes: part road trip diary, part name-dropping celebrity exposé, part long-winded *Braveheart* metaphor. One look at the sales records will tell you that those are the sorts of meditation books many people would like to read, as most of us "fidgety skeptics" can relate to his frustrations and disillusionment (if not his glamorous lifestyle).

Mindful Running: How Meditative Running Can Improve Your Performance and Make You a Happier, More Fulfilled Person by Mackenzie L. Havey.
New York: Bloomsbury, 2017. ISBN 978-1-4729-4486-3; Paperback; US$14.00/Can$19.00.

Runners are always looking for books to improve their performance. The next time someone walks in looking for your running books, hand them this. While I can't guarantee it will make them a "happier, more fulfilled person," the tips and tricks in here will certainly make their running (and obsessing about running) more enjoyable, which is all any of us runners can really hope for. Once they finish this one, offer them *Running with the Mind of Meditation: Lessons for Training Body and Mind* (Harmony, 2013) by Sakyong Mipham, which I prefer but is sprinkled with a bit more Buddhist dogma, so not to everyone's taste.

Not Always So: Practicing the True Spirit of Zen by Shunryu Suzuki.
New York: HarperCollins, 2002. ISBN 978-0-0601-9785-8; Hardcover; US$22.95/Can$34.95.

Suzuki Roshi was most famous for his classic *Zen Mind, Beginner's Mind*, but this lesser-known assemblage of his lectures is also a valuable addition to any dedicated meditation collection. The Roshi's teaching methods are through parables and also simple admonishments to continue sitting. Just sitting. Not suppressing or inviting thoughts or sensations, just sitting. And when we feel ourselves becoming attached, digging in our heels, obsessing, flailing about on the open seas of life, he reminds us that everything is in a constant state of flux, and also nothing changes. "Don't stick to anything," reminds the Roshi, "not even the truth." Because the truth, like everything, is *not always so*.

Unplug: A Simple Guide to Meditation for Busy Skeptics and Modern Soul Seekers by Suze Yalof Schwartz and Debra Goldstein.
New York: Harmony Books, 2017. ISBN 978-1-101-90536-4; Hardcover; US$22.99/Can$29.99.

When they say this guide is simple, they mean it. Written in a friendly tone, Yalof Schwartz speaks to the reader from personal experience of how meditation has changed her life for the better. She equates it with going to the gym: it's only for a few minutes a day, but if you keep doing it consistently, you'll see the results. She frames our "monkey mind" as "Google brain," which many readers in this digital age can relate to. We have all these tabs open, all these alerts streaming in, but with meditation we can choose to close the tabs, drag the thoughts that are spam to the trash folder, and put our devices on airplane mode. Gentle cheerleading combined with basic instruction makes this a great book to have in your collection and put in the hands of readers just starting out on their meditation journey.

Yoga for Healthy Aging: A Guide to Lifelong Well-Being by Baxter Bell and Nina Zolotow.
Boulder, CO: Shambhala, 2017. ISBN 978-1-61180-385-3; Paperback; US$24.95/Can$33.95.

The average human life span is around seventy-nine years and the aging process is something no one escapes (despite our very best efforts!). How we treat our bodies during those give-or-take seventy-nine years greatly impacts the quality of our lives and how we feel living in those bodies. The field of gerontology has emerged to study the aging process—which is incredibly complex—and the authors of this excellent book posit that by focusing on three essential concepts we can age healthily: compressed morbidity (short periods of time in ill health), independence (having physical, financial, and mental freedom), and equanimity (emotional and physical resilience). Guess what helps with all three of those things? Yoga and meditation! The first half of the book focuses on the theory behind why we practice, how it relates to healthy aging, and how to adapt the poses to your own particularities. The second half of the book is filled with a wonderful, comprehensive selection of sequences and individual poses with many variations. This book is highly recommended as an addition to your circulating collection but also to teach from.

SUGGESTIONS FOR PROFESSIONAL DEVELOPMENT COLLECTION

Teaching Yoga: Essential Foundations and Techniques by Mark Stephens.
Berkeley, CA: North Atlantic Books, 2010. ISBN 978-1-55643-885-1; Paperback; US$22.95/Can$26.95.

This manual covers everything the modern yoga teacher-in-training could need to know before starting to teach. It begins with a history of yoga and how contemporary *Hatha* styles developed and evolved. It goes over energy work, anatomy, how to set up a room for teaching, modifications, and how to use props. There are scripts for how to cue physical poses, how to sequence a class, and how to work with those who have special needs, such as pregnant students or those with injuries. *Pranayama* (breathing) exercises, as well as meditation, are also thoroughly addressed. It even has a chapter on how to create a yoga business, which has helpful hints for library staff about how to market programs. For those of us who are already certified, the book serves as a great ready-reference for *Asanas*, as it contains a large table at the back, listing them in alphabetical order by their Sanskrit name (with pronunciation key and common English names). The chart also includes black-and-white photos of each pose. There are more in-depth explorations of each pose in chapter 7, including contraindications for each pose. An excellent addition to the professional development collection, and would also be appreciated in the circulating collection by those patrons undergoing yoga teacher training, or considering it.

I Don't Want To, I Don't Feel Like It: How Resistance Controls Your Life and What to Do about It by Cheri Huber and Ashwini Narayanan.
Murphys, CA: Keep It Simple Press, 2013. ISBN 978-0-9614754-9-9; Paperback; US$12.00/Can$13.86.

At first glance this book doesn't seem to have much to do with meditation, but once you open its cover you'll discover it is steeped in Zen teachings. Unassuming and, frankly, horribly produced, this is a mediocre resource to get the trepidatious inquirer interested in mindfulness. It is most useful for the teaching librarian for its chapter called "Tools for Garden Living: A 30-Day Retreat," which contains stories and exercises for the novice to ponder and practice. One, for example, explores the concept of *Gassho*, which is bringing the hands together at the heart and bowing. It goes beyond that and teaches of the method of living in *Gassho*, which is an acceptance of, and reverence for, the interconnection of all living things. It does this by telling the story of how the meditation teacher explains to their pupils that cultivating an attitude of habitual reverence is like filling a sieve with water. When we try to pour water cup by cup into the sieve, it flows through to the other side. But if we throw the sieve into the ocean, it submerges and sinks to the bottom, as we too must throw ourselves into the service of a life of *Gassho* and not dole out little cupfuls of practice into an otherwise ego-driven existence. Heavy stuff for a modest little book with childlike hand-drawn illustrations and off-putting faux-handwriting font (its major downfall). For its price, it is worth grabbing some stories out of for programs, but not an easy read on the eyes. Patrons might not be as picky if you'd like to add it to your circulating collection, but I would keep it for use among library staff.

Yoga Adjustments: Philosophy, Principles, and Techniques by Mark Stephens. Berkeley, CA: North Atlantic Books, 2014. ISBN 978-1-58394-770-8; Paperback; US$24.95/Can$28.95.

While our comfort levels, policies, patrons, or training may not allow us to do any hands-on assists while instructing a yoga class at our library, this helpful guide offers many verbal cues that can be given (along with pictures for every adjustment) to guide our students into better alignment. It also offers modifications with props, like straps and blocks, which can be incredible assets in a teacher's arsenal. In addition to those, for those who do want to offer hands-on assists, Stephens addresses the ethical concerns of touching our students and gives seven essential principals for using touch in class. A must-read for every yogi-librarian.

Yoga Sequencing: Designing Transformative Yoga Classes by Mark Stephens. Berkeley, CA: North Atlantic Books, 2012. ISBN 978-1-58394-497-4; Paperback; US$24.95/Can$28.95.

This essential guide by popular and prolific author Mark Stephens is the perfect companion to any yoga teacher, no matter their lineage, ability, or length of time teaching. It gets so much play in my teaching and personal practice that I've had the spine removed and hole-punched all 507 pages and put it in a giant binder for ease of use. With sixty-seven sequences and more than two thousand photos, this manual is the go-to guide for how to design a yoga class. It goes beyond the basic arc structure outlined in Stephens's *Teaching Yoga* to create anatomy-focused classes for beginner, intermediate, and advanced students. There are also special sequences and advice for teaching children (elementary, middle, and high school classes), menstruation, pregnancy, and post-natal (including special classes for each trimester), menopause, preventing osteoporosis, reducing mood swings, and seniors. There is even an appendix of popular methods, such as Iyengar or Kripalu. A must-have for every professional collection that supports libraries that have yoga programs.[4]

Key Points

- When offering yoga and meditation to adults and seniors, remember they have busy lives, especially those juggling family responsibilities. Offer programs at various time slots to accommodate work schedules. Be mindful of offering modifications for those of differing abilities.
- Program models can be altered to fit with the library's hours of operation and staff availability, and can also be used as outreach initiatives. These are all low-budget programs.
- Try to make displays of materials to correspond with events to promote literacy and increase circulation.
- Collection development of yoga and meditation materials for adults and seniors is important, and there are many resources on the market for both the general public and for professional use. Share them widely.

1. See www.jenncarson.com/resources.html.

2. Lordo Rinzler, "10 Blunt Truths about Becoming a Meditation Teacher," *Elephant Journal*, July 21, 2015, https://www.elephantjournal.com/2015/07/10-blunt-truths-about-becoming-a-meditation-teacher/.

3. Thich Nhat Hanh, *Making Space: Creating a Home Meditation Practice* (Berkeley, CA: Parallax, 2001).

4. A different version of this review first appeared on www.yoganthelibrary.com.

CHAPTER 11

Yoga for Every *Body*: Inclusive Programming through Outreach and Inreach

The Importance of Outreach

IF YOU HAVE THE MEANS and the resources to be able to reach out to your community beyond the four walls of your library, I highly suggest you do it. Many books have been written on the subject of library outreach for good reason: it is an excellent way to get new patrons interested in the library and it breaks down often invisible barriers that may have prevented certain demographics of patrons from accessing your services (for example, those with misinformed beliefs that library programs cost money, or patrons lacking transportation means, or those who are wary of government institutions). Movement-based

OUTREACH OPPORTUNITIES

Here is a list of possible outreach opportunities that may work in your community; feel free to add to it, this is simply a jumping-off point.

- After-school programs
- Airports and train stations
- Banks
- Bookmobile and book bike programs
- Bookstores
- Business associations
- Churches and religious groups
- Community and civic centers
- Day cares and preschools
- Digital services: podcasts/webinars/ meet-ups/videos
- Employment centers
- Festivals
- Funeral homes
- Garden clubs
- Gyms and fitness clubs
- Head Start
- Homeless shelters
- Homeschool associations
- Hospitals
- Juvenile detention centers
- Knitting/art/craft groups
- Malls
- Multicultural/immigrant centers and programs
- Museums and heritage centers
- Nursing or compassionate care homes
- Occupational therapy clinics
- Parks, playgrounds, and beaches
- Prisons and county jails
- Recovery centers
- Rotary clubs and other social groups
- Schools and alternative schools
- Scouts/Guides
- Sports groups
- Student lounges or commons (for academic librarians)
- Tourist or visitor information centers
- Town hall
- Wellness and health centers
- Women's shelters
- Zoos

outreach, such as yoga, or mindfulness-based outreach, such as meditation, is also an excellent opportunity to reach underserved populations who could especially benefit from these programs. And don't think of outreach as only being a library staffer visiting a location in the community; outreach can also be done online or over the phone through promoting digital services and resources.

◎ The Importance of Inreach

While we spend a great deal of time and energy trying to promote wellness programs to patrons (and hoping to snag the attention of potential patrons) we forget to take care of ourselves and each other. Librarians and library staff experience a high rate of burnout and work-related stress. As Kelly Starrett reminds us in his excellent book *Deskbound: Standing Up to a Sitting World*, "The typical seated office worker has more musculoskeletal injuries than any other industry sector worker, including construction, metal industry, and transportation workers."[1] In other words, we have *more* injuries to our muscles and bones than people who *do manual labor*. Some of the ramifications of sitting at a computer all day include neck pain, carpal tunnel syndrome, an increased risk of heart disease, TMJ disorder, pelvic floor dysfunction, weight gain, and soreness in the hips, chest, and shoulders. Listening to my colleagues complain about their ailments for the last decade, I wouldn't hesitate to assume that most library staff have experienced at least one of these conditions. I know I have, and I work at a standing desk at least half my workday, exercise six to seven days a week, and lead an otherwise healthy lifestyle. As Starrett maintains in *Deskbound*, working out, even for more than an hour a day, isn't enough to counteract all the negative repetitive strain and sedentary habits we regularly engage in, year after year after year. Our bodies want to be in motion. And our bodies also crave rest and silence. One of the biggest issues my staff at the public library complain about is being constantly interrupted: by patrons, by the ringing phone, by mail deliveries, by emails, by each other . . . which is all part of the job but which makes it easy to make clerical errors, lose your train of thought, and generally just feel scattered and overwhelmed. When planning your program calendar don't forget to include meditation and yoga breaks for your staff. Here's some ways you can incorporate more mindfulness into their days (and yours!):

- Encourage staff to take stretch breaks by hanging yoga posters in the break room or in work areas. You can download a free *De-stress at Your Desk* poster complete with fifteen-minute yoga routine at http://www.jenncarson.com/assets/de-stress_ at_your_desk_english.pdf.
- Encourage staff self-care by sharing this free poster called *Taking Care of Us* at http://www.jenncarson.com/assets/taking_care_of_us.pdf or watching my *Taking Care of Us* webinar created for the American Library Association: http://program-minglibrarian.org/learn/taking-care-us-ergonomic-advice-library-staff.
- Encourage yoga or stretch breaks during staff meetings or training.
- During conferences or training days set aside a "quiet room" that people can go to in order to eat, meditate, or rest in silence. There should be no talking or devices allowed in the room (tapping buttons or typing can be distracting or irritating to those who are experiencing sensory overload).
- Set a timer on your phone to ring every thirty or sixty minutes to remind you to take a short mindfulness or stretch break.

Program Models for Outreach and Inreach

The following pages will offer a variety of programs designed to serve exceptional populations. Four of these classes can be modified for use inside the library or out in the community, and one introduces an opportunity to connect with patrons virtually. Teddy Bear Yoga (page 129) is designed for children on the autism spectrum or with other sensory processing disorders. Online Mindfulness Meet-Up (page 135) teaches patrons how to meditate over the internet. Day Care Yoga Storytime (page 137) promotes mindful movement and literacy services to caregivers and children. Chair Yoga for Lifelong Health (page 140) is designed for patrons with limited mobility or for staff or other office workers to use at their desks. Lastly, there is Yoga for Heartache (page 145), a chance to offer a movement-based mindfulness program to community members who may be experiencing grief or recovering from trauma.

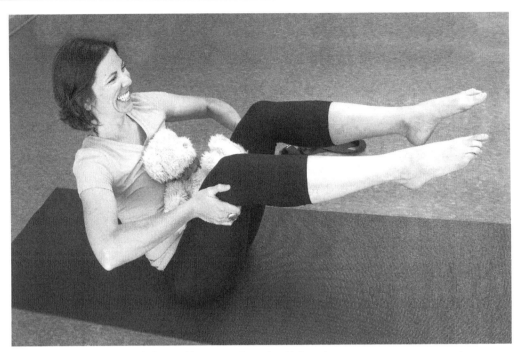

Figure 11.1. Even teddy bears like yoga. *Brendan Helmuth*

A program for your young patrons who may be too scared or shy to try yoga on their own, but can bring their teddy bear (or *lovely*, or *stuffy*, or whatever they call it) along for emotional support. This is a great program to market to families who have children on the autism spectrum or other sensory processing disorders. It is low key, low risk, and low stimulation. Many children with characteristics associated with autism have impaired social skills, difficulty with anxiety, low muscle tone, and limited body awareness. They usually associate being told to be quiet with something punitive, but this program reinforces that sitting still and learning to self-soothe is a healthy skill. As Louise Goldberg affirms in *Yoga Therapy for Children with Autism and Special Needs*, yoga levels the playing field between adults and children.[2] We get down on our hands and knees and use the universal languages of touch, breath, and movement. The best part? Teddy bears are *great* at doing yoga. They can take over doing the poses when your little yogis need a sensory break. Teddy bears are also great at listening to stories! You are going to read the students a picture book at the end of the program, and then they are going to read stories to their teddies.

Advance Planning

Step 1. Find a teacher that has a CCYT designation (certified children's yoga teacher) and preferably one who has experience teaching kids with exceptionalities. Try your local occupational therapy clinic or autism outreach group for leads. Or if you have the necessary background yourself, feel free to teach the class. For example, I am a CCYT, but also am trained as an autism support worker and used to work as an interventionist with kids who had behavioral issues in the schools. So I feel confident in my skill set. You will need to exude a calm, empathetic, quiet confidence for this program to be most effective.

Step 2. Pick a day and time for the event. Take into account the age range you want to offer it to. If you want to include elementary-age children, an after-school or week-end time slot may be best. If you are aiming for preschoolers, a weekday morning may be great. Or anytime during summer vacation. The program should last no more than forty-five minutes, with lots of room for contingencies and no program planned directly afterward so people aren't made to rush out of the room and can stay for some free play.

Step 3. Decide whether this will be a one-off program or an ongoing weekly or monthly event. Perhaps try it out once and see how it is received and then decide whether or not to offer it again. You also need to decide if it is going to be drop-in or registration only.

Step 4. Book the room you will be using. Space may play a factor in how many people can attend. The quietest room in the library, with dimmable lights, and easy access to a washroom is best. If your expected patrons are regular library users, have it in a room you know they are already familiar with and comfortable.

Step 5. Make sure you have all the required materials (see list below).

Step 6. Advertise your event if you are offering on-site. Make a print poster. Make a Facebook event. Put it on your website and event calendar. Tweet about it. Visit local day cares and schools and autism support centers to drop off a poster for families to see. Don't forget about homeschool families! If you are offering out in the community, only advertise if it is available to the general public and not for a specific group. If that is the case, allow them to control the registration process.

Step 7. Do the paperwork. Make a sign-up sheet if you require registration. Prepare liability waivers. I don't recommend taking photos during the event, even though it is nice to document what you are doing. The less distracting or anxiety-provoking stimuli, the better.

Step 8. Acquire a copy of *Hug Me, Please!* by Przemyslaw Wechterowicz.[3] Read it a few times to familiarize yourself with the story. This is the tale of Little Bear and Daddy Bear who spend the day going through the forest hugging everyone they come across: a beaver, a weasel, even the Big Bad Wolf and a hunter, and more! Everyone they encounter is changed in some way by their affectionate intervention, even the bears themselves who decide they really enjoy all the hugging. Then Little Bear realizes the only creatures in the forest they forgot to hug were each other.

Step 9. Look over the infographic (see pages 133–134) to familiarize yourself with the sequence or share with the teacher you've recruited (or they may have a sequence of their own they'd rather use).

Materials Required

- Storybooks geared to your age group, with a variety of reading levels
- Yoga mats
- Extra teddy bears
- Singing bowl or bell
- Optional, but nice: a visual timer so students can see when class starts and ends (I like the ones made by Time Timers brand)
- Coloring sheets (of teddy bears) and crayons or markers on a table off to the side for those who need a break from participating
- Liability waivers and clipboard
- *Hug Me, Please!* by Przemyslaw Wechterowicz

Budget Details

$0–$200. If you already have yoga mats and a couple of teddy bears on hand (or ones borrowed from home), this program can be done at pretty much no cost. Especially if you don't need to hire a teacher (or can find one who would volunteer). You may be able to apply for funding through autism advocacy groups or other accessibility support services.

Day of Event

Step 1. Prepare the room by setting out the mats, coloring table, timer, and books. Get your waivers and clipboard ready.

Step 2. Greet your patrons, have the parents/guardians sign a waiver, and invite them to have a seat on one of the mats and get comfortable.

Step 3. Explain clearly what is going to happen. Like any children's program, establish ground rules at the beginning. Here are some suggestions:

- Rule 1. When you hear *this* noise (ding the bell, or whatever you are using), please return to the top of your mat and sit in Easy Pose (or crisscross applesauce, as I call it).
- Rule 2. Keep your hands to yourself during class and stay on your own mat unless asked to do otherwise.
- Rule 3. Only do what feels good for your body. If something doesn't feel good, sit on your mat in Easy Pose and practice your belly breathing until the next pose.

Step 4: Have each child sit in a circle with their teddy bear or stuffy on their lap. Read *Hug Me, Please!* When you are done the story ask the students how they felt about the bears giving everyone hugs. Ask them to share whether they like to be hugged, and if they do, by whom (strangers, family members, their parents, a special friend) and who they like to hug the most (sometimes who we like to hug and who we like to be hugged by can be different). If some people in the group say they don't like hugs, tell them that is totally OK! Ask them if there was anyone in the story who didn't like hugs either. Ask them if they think it is OK to hug someone who doesn't want to be hugged (great opportunity to talk about the importance of consent and safe touch in an age-appropriate way). Ask them if they like to hug their teddies or stuffies or pillows instead of people.

Step 5. Follow along with the infographic, skipping poses that are too challenging or shortening the sequence depending on the age and abilities of your audience.

Step 6. After class, give everyone some time to free play with the blocks and straps or do a coloring page. Many will want to try to ring your bell or singing bowl.

Step 7. Thank everyone for coming and ask them to help you put away the props (good team-building activity and gives sense of ownership and contribution).

Advice

- I like to have a whiteboard with the poses and activities written in order on it. Then as each pose/activity is completed, you can invite one of the young patrons to come wipe it off the board or cross it out. This gives them a sense of control over what is going to happen next and a sense of accomplishment at completing tasks.

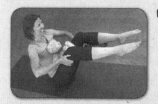

TEDDY BEAR YOGA

Here's a fun routine for little yogis that may be too scared or shy to try yoga on their own but can bring their teddy bear along for emotional support. It is low-key, low-risk, and low-stimulation. We get down on our hands and knees and use the universal languages of touch, breath, and movement. The best part? Teddy bears are great at doing yoga, so they can take over when you need a sensory break!

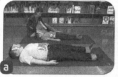 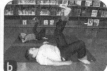 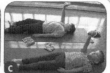

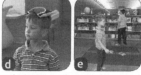

1. Bean Bag Balance (a) Have the student lie on a mat. Place a bean bag on the student's belly. Their teddy bear can sit on top of the bean bag if they'd like. Have them notice that the bean bag goes up when they breathe in and goes down when they breathe out. (b) Try balancing the bean bag on each foot. (c) Try balancing the bean bag on each hand. (d) Try balancing the bean bag on the head while standing. (e) Try balancing the bean bag while walking.

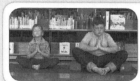

3. Butterfly Have the child sit with their feet touching and knees bent to the side. If it is more comfortable, they can place a block under each knee for support. Have them bring their hands to heart center and close their eyes. Take 5 deep breaths.

2. Lion's Breath Sitting in an easy crossed-leg position, have the child take a very deep breath and scrunch up their face and make fists with their hands, tightening their whole bodies. Then have them breathe out hard and stick out their tongues and spread their fingers wide. This helps release tension in their bodies. Repeat 3 times. They can also do this lying on their back or sitting in a chair.

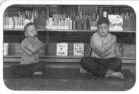

4. Self-Hug Have the child cross their arms over their chest and give themselves a hug. Ask them to try squeezing harder or softer to discover what level of pressure they like. Have them give their teddy bears a hug. Ask them if their teddy bears like soft, medium, or hard hugs.

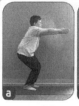

5. Bow and Arrow (a) Have the child stand with their feet touching. Have them bend their knees and raise their arms in the air in front of their chest. (b) Have them make a fist with their right hand, take a deep breath in, and bend their arm back like they are pulling on a bow string, looking over their right shoulder. Then they exhale and release their arm, shooting it forward like an arrow. Repeat with the left arm. Then repeat 4 more times each side. If they get tired from squatting, let them do it standing.

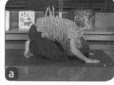 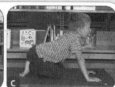

6. Rabbit (a) Have the child come into a kneeling position with their toes curled under and their head on the floor. If they don't like their toes curled, they can be flat. (b) Have them reach back and touch their feet. You can apply gentle pressure on their lower back if they like this. Some will find it soothing; others won't. (c) Have them come forward on their hands and stick out their tongue. This helps release tension.

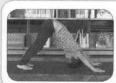

7. Down Dog Have the child push into their feet and stick their hips in the air, coming into an inverted V position. They can shake their head from side to side to release tension in the neck. Take 5 breaths and then lower the knees to the floor.

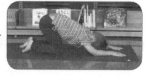

8. Child's Pose From the kneeling position have the child lower their head to the ground and round their spine, lowering their seat to their feet if possible. Take 5 breaths

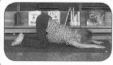

9. Puppy Have the child straighten their back and lift their hips in the air, pressing down through their hands, forehead resting on the mat. Take 5 breaths.

10. Frog Have the child lower down like a frog squatting on its hind legs. Ask them to balance by lifting their hands off the mat and holding their knees. They can also hold their teddy bear for an extra challenge. Their heels can be planted on the mat or lifted. Take 5 breaths.

Figure 11.2.

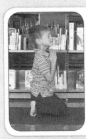

11. Toe Stretch From a kneeling position, have the child curl their toes under and sit back toward their heels. If they find this uncomfortable, they can try placing a rolled up mat between their thighs and their calves. Take 5 breaths.

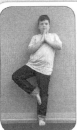

12. Tree From a standing position have the child raise the right foot to their left ankle, calf, or thigh. They can lean against a wall for support. They can bring their hands to heart center or raise their arms overhead like branches. Take 5 breaths and then lower the foot and repeat on the left side.

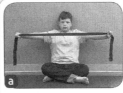

13. Strap Stretch (a) Have the child hold a strap or belt in their hands as far apart as is comfortable for their shoulders. Take 5 breaths. (b) Have the child reach their arms overhead, leaning against a wall for support if necessary. Take 5 breaths. (c) Lean the arms and torso to one side and then the other. Take 5 breaths.

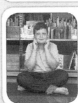

14. Ear Pull Have the child reach up and find their earlobes. Have them take a deep breath and gently pull down. Ask them if they like the sensation. Ask them to gently pull on the other parts of the ears while taking deep breaths. This is very soothing for the nervous system and helps them with sensory self-regulation. Now it's the teddy bear's turn. Be gentle!

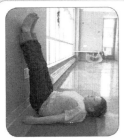

15. Legs Up the Wall Have the child lie on their back with their legs up the wall. They can also lie on the floor with their knees bent at a 90° angle and their calves resting on a chair. Their arms can be at their sides or out wide in a T shape. Take 5 breaths.

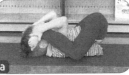

16. Happy Baby (a) Have the child lie on their back and bring their knees toward their chest. Have them reach their arms between their legs and hold their own feet. Take 5 breaths. (b) For more of a challenge, they can lower their knees to the floor and reach their hands toward their lower backs.

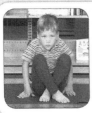

18. Uplifting Pose From a cross-legged position, have the child place their hands on the mat next to their hips. Option to place blocks under their hands for comfort. Have them lift their knees toward their chin and press into their hands, lifting their seat off the ground.

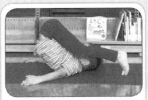

17. Plow Have the child lie on their back and rock their hips forward, bringing their toes over their head. They can lower their toes toward the floor or rest them on a block. Their hands can rest on the mat or come to their lower back.

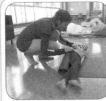
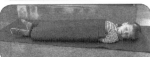

19. Burrito Have the child lie across the mat, with their feet and head off the surface of it. Gently roll them up in the mat, applying an even amount of pressure. Once they are all rolled up, have them close their eyes and breathe in and out through their nose. For those that don't like the Burrito, they can lie in traditional *Savasana*.

20. Storytime Read the child a story such as *Hug Me, Please!* by Przemyslaw Wechterowicz, *I Am Yoga* by Susan Verde, or *Knuffle Bunny* by Mo Willems. Then they can practice reading a story to their teddy bear, a friend, or a sibling. If the child isn't reading yet, they can explain what is happening from looking at the pictures.

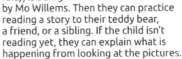

Jenn Carson is a physical literacy expert, yoga instructor, librarian, and the author of *Get Your Community Moving: Physical Literacy Programs for All Ages.*

Program design by Jenn Carson • Photography by Karen Ruet • Layout by Brendan Helmuth

Figure 11.3.

- Keep your numbers low. Too many kids makes for too much noise and overstimulation for everyone (especially you).
- The number of poses accomplished and the length of time each one is held is irrelevant here. Same goes for getting "proper" technique. We're just encouraging the students to try something new and reap the physical and mental benefits from yoga breathing and the postures. Feeling safe and accepted is more important than number of poses accomplished or perfect execution.
- Remember, children on the autism spectrum may appear indifferent or listen without affect (no visibly emotional reaction), but this doesn't mean they aren't absorbing what is being said and processing it in their own ways.
- Under- or over-responsiveness to touch and sound is common for children with autism spectrum disorder (ASD) and other sensory processing disorders. Don't be surprised if you get wildly different reactions from each child during the practice.
- You may end up with a child who has attention deficit hyperactivity disorder (ADHD) in the same room as kids with ASD because families often bring siblings to class together and you can't exactly refuse non-ASD students or even neurotypical siblings, since that wouldn't be very inclusive. Children with ADHD often fidget, have difficulty focusing on one task at a time, talk frequently, and are challenged by turn taking or waiting for instruction. You can counter this—and put everyone at ease—by repeating instructions clearly and often, breaking each pose down into small tasks, and offering small rewards upon task completion (such as getting to cross the name of the pose off the whiteboard).
- Are you a librarian-yogi in a high school or interested in offering this sort of program to an older audience? Take out the teddies and instead do Fidget Spinner Yoga. Your students can bring their favorite fidget device, which can be used as a focus point during the class, and then they can build their own fidget spinners after using Legos or other supplies. Search online for "build your own fidget spinner" tutorials for ideas!
- Consider having a coloring table or some sort of sensory bin available for those who need a break (and need to be given a break) from participating. They can rejoin the group when and if they feel ready.

⊚ Program Model: Online Mindfulness Meet-Up

This thirty-minute online program is an opportunity to reach those with limited access to transportation—or limited mobility—but who can use digital devices from home. The relative anonymity of the platform may encourage people with social anxiety or sensory processing issues to access the services and join in the conversation at their own discretion or in a way that may feel more comfortable for them.

Advance Planning

Step 1. Set the date and time for your first session. Think about your target audience (working professionals? students? seniors?) and then pick the best time/date (evenings? noon? weekday mornings?).

Step 2. Find a free online meet-up software like Zoom or Google Hangouts and make sure to do a test run a day or two before the event. Have a staff member try to log in from their device for troubleshooting. Make sure your mic and webcam work.

Step 3. Gather all necessary materials (see "Materials Required" below).

Step 4. Advertise. You can promote the meet-up through your library's social media channels, website, program calendar, and perhaps even a print poster in your branch or community. Make sure to take advantage of word-of-mouth advertising by mentioning the program at the reference and circulation desk to anyone who comes in seeking information on the topic, and in programs where you think patrons may be receptive.

Materials Required

- Meet-up software
- Singing bowl, chime, or bell on your phone
- Timer, on your phone, computer, or watch

Budget Details

$0. This program shouldn't cost anything to run, since you are using free software and your existing work computer and timer.

Day of Event

Here's an example of what an online mindfulness meet-up might look like.

Step 1. Introduce yourself and any other staff members who are joining you and thank everyone for joining. Depending on the size of the meet-up, you may wish to have everyone go around and introduce themselves (works well with eight or fewer people), or jump right in.

Step 2. Explain what mindfulness is, which is basically the ability to recognize what is going on in your mind, body, and surroundings, without getting caught up by it. So for example, you may hear the fridge humming, or feel hungry, or have a thought about your best friend, or feel irritated, but you don't get caught up in any of it. You just use the practice of *noticing* the thought, sensation, or environmental input, and then you look at it with a sort of friendly curiosity, without judgment. Like, "Huh, look at that, I'm thinking about waffles." I like using the common teaching metaphor of the sky, and how are thoughts are like clouds—sometimes stormy and threatening, sometimes cute little puffballs, sometimes murky fog—but we can just watch them go by; we don't have to let the weather ruin our day.

Step 3. After you have explained what mindfulness is, open the floor to allow for any questions or clarification.

Step 4. Invite everyone to join in for a mindfulness exercise together. Ask them to notice where they are in this moment, and see if they can describe it to themselves (in their heads) in a very straightforward way, without judgment. For example, "I am sitting in my favorite chair. My feet are planted on the floor and the sun is shining in the room" or "I am walking through the park with my phone in my hand and the breeze is cool" or "I am lying on the floor next to my laptop. The carpet is soft."

Step 5. Now ask them to notice how their bodies are feeling, by doing a scan of their bodies from their toes to the top of their head. Guide them through this, using a script that runs along these lines: "I am noticing my toes. I give my toes a little wiggle. I am noticing my ankles, how my ankles feel. I am noticing my calves, my knees, the backs of my knees. Now I am noticing my thighs and hips . . ." and so forth.

Step 6. Now invite them to notice their breath. Ask them to feel the coolness of the breath as it enters the nostrils, and feel the gentle warmth of the breath as it leaves. Have them continue to follow the breath as it moves in and out of the nose, and notice the belly as it rises and falls. If they find their mind wandering off while doing this exercise, remind them that is totally normal and to be expected, and to bring their mind back to their breath. And when it wanders away again, without judgment, like noticing the clouds in the sky, label the thought as "thinking" and then come back to the breath. Perhaps they will experience the distraction of an internal sensation or external disruption, in which case they can be encouraged to label that too, such as "hunger" or "itching" or "dog barking" and then come back to the breath. Tell them you are going to set a timer for five minutes and have everyone stay on the line and continue this practice silently, together, until you ring the bell to bring them out.

Advice

- Make sure to have a second event planned so that at the end of the first one (which will hopefully be well attended) you will have a date you can share with the attendees.
- Make sure, if you leave time for Q&A at the end, that you finish on time and watch the clock (unless you want to keep it open ended, but people (especially if you had a large audience) may talk for quite a while!
- That said, don't be too disappointed if you only get one or two people for your first meet-up. Or no one. Maybe it was the timing. Maybe not enough people knew about it. Try to spread the word during your other wellness-type programs, or to anyone who checks out a book on mindfulness or meditation, or try it to a specific audience where you already have an in, such as a community college class your colleague is teaching, or to a group of staff members in another branch.

◎ Program Model: Day Care Yoga Storytime

Sometimes it is really difficult for day care groups to get to the library for programs, depending on traffic, timetables, liability worries, lack of transportation, and more. So why not go to them and show them what the library can offer? Bring along flyers and print calendars to send home with the kids to make sure parents know what's on offer during evenings and weekends. Make sure to bring along some fun sensory toys from the library. Add some yoga moves and mindfulness to your storytime and—voila!—you've got a physical literacy party happening! This program will last thirty to forty-five minutes.

Advance Planning

Step 1. Pick what day care or after-school center you'd like to approach, call them to explain what you are offering, and see if you can agree on a mutually beneficial date and time.

Step 2. Ask the day care how much space they have available, how many children will be attending, and the ages. Rather than lug yoga mats and/or meditation cushions all

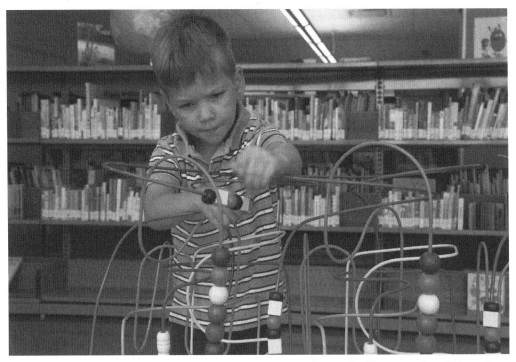

Figure 11.4. Day cares can visit your library or you can bring the library to them! *Karen Ruet*

over town, see if the day care already has cushions for the children to sit on (sometimes referred to as "sit-upons" in the biz), or chairs, and plan a program that can be done in tight quarters. If they have lots of open space and you want to bring mats, use one of the programs outlined in chapter 7 (for preschoolers) or chapter 8 (for the after-school crowd). The program model below is designed for no mats, preschool age, and a small classroom space.

Step 3. Check with your administration and the day care to confirm you are covered for injury and/or liability in case you or someone in the class gets injured. It's always a good idea to print off liability waivers and have the parents sign ahead of time, or the caregivers from the day care if that is deemed acceptable.

Step 4. Before the event, gather all the necessary materials (see "Materials Required" below).

Step 5. Read through the storybooks you will be using (*Meditate with Me: A Step-by-Step Mindfulness Journey* by Mariam Gates and Margarita Surnaite and *You Are a Lion! And Other Fun Yoga Poses* by Taeeun Yoo) and familiarize yourself with the exercises.

Materials Required

- Liability waivers
- Photo release forms, if planning on taking pictures
- Singing bowl or bell or gong
- Adult-size cushion for you to use, if you prefer that to a chair
- Meditation picture book (*Meditate with Me: A Step-by-Step Mindfulness Journey* by Mariam Gates and Margarita Surnaite is the one used in this program model, but there are many other options listed in chapter 8)
- Yoga picture book (*You Are a Lion! And Other Fun Yoga Poses* by Taeeun Yoo is the one used in this program model, but there are many other options listed in chapter 8)

- Blank paper and crayons (the day care may supply these—double-check—or you can bring your own)
- A jar full of water and glitter
- A balloon

Budget Details

$0–$50. This program can be done very cheaply. You will need to purchase a copy of *You Are a Lion! And Other Fun Yoga Poses* by Taeeun Yoo (US$17.99) and *Meditate with Me: A Step-by-Step Mindfulness Journey* by Mariam Gates and Margarita Surnaite (US$17.99), if you don't already have them in your library system (or borrow through ILL!). You will need some sort of bell (even if you just use a free app on your phone to keep costs down), and the other craft supplies you probably already have on hand.

Day of Event

Step 1. Introduce yourself to the group and tell everyone that you are there from the library to read them some stories and learn a little bit about yoga and mindfulness. Ask the class if they have ever tried yoga before (many probably have!). Is it like stretching? Is it like dancing? Is it like playing pretend animals? Ask them to show you their favorite pose if they have one (the ones who don't will do something silly anyway). Ask them if they know what mindfulness is. Ask them what they think the difference is between a mind and a brain. Ask them what they think thoughts are made of. Be prepared for some very inventive and interesting answers!

Step 2. Have everyone gather on a spot on the floor (wherever they do circle time). A circle is good, just make sure there is a bit of space between them. Explain that the rule during the storytime is: if they hear the singing bowl/bell/gong they are to come back to sitting in crisscross applesauce (Easy Pose) on their spot with their hands on their thighs (ring the bell to demonstrate). Let them start fidgeting and then ring it again. They will love this. Tell them you are going to read them a story about yoga and do some poses along with the kids in the story (*You Are a Lion!* features preschool-age kids, so it is perfect). Ask them if they know what *Namaste* means. Tell them it means that all the good in me says hello to all the good in you. Have them practice saying *Namaste* to each other and to you with their hands folded together in the center of their chest (Prayer Pose). Show them the picture of the little girl on the first page with her hands at heart center and say, "Whenever we hear the word *Namaste* in the book, we'll do this with our hands and say it together! It's a nice way to tell people you care about them. Then we're going to follow along and do the different poses in the book, so spread out your arms in a circle and make sure you have a bit of space around you so you won't hit your neighbors."

Step 3. Read *You Are a Lion! And Other Fun Yoga Poses* and act out the poses along with the kids, ending with *Namaste* and lying on the floor in *Savasana* (Corpse Pose). Ring the singing bowl/bell/gong to bring everyone out and back into crisscross applesauce (Easy Pose).

Step 4. Have everyone grab a kid-size chair and sit with their feet flat on the floor and their hands in their laps. If their classroom doesn't have chairs, do the next step sitting on cushions on the floor in crisscross applesauce pose.

Step 5. Read *Meditate with Me: A Step-by-Step Mindfulness Journey* and follow along with the instructions. Be prepared to shake a glitter jar, show mad/happy/excited/sad with your whole body (not the easiest thing to do even for grown-ups!), and blow up a balloon.

Step 6. When you get to the page of the book where it cues everyone to close their eyes (the page has animals sitting on chairs in a class with their eyes closed), ask the kids to close their eyes while you read the last few pages (turn the book toward you so they are less likely to peek because they want to see the pictures). When you get to the last page, pause for a few minutes and let silence fill the room (hopefully—it's hard with pre-schoolers!), and then ring your singing bowl/bell/gong to bring them out of the silence and back to crisscross applesauce. If they were on chairs it will be fun to see if they jump down to the floor or if they try to do the pose on the chair!

Step 7. Remind the children how they learned in the story that their mind is like the sky, and the thoughts are the clouds drifting by. Have them take out their paper and crayons and draw their internal sky for you. Is it stormy? Are there big clouds? Little puffballs? Fog? Sunshine? Talk about how the weather changes and never stays the same for too long. Ask them how they feel when the sun comes out after a storm, or how they feel on a rainy day. Let them chatter while they work on their pictures and then, if there is time, give everyone the opportunity to share at the end.

Step 8. Thank everyone for going on your yoga adventure together and leave behind some flyers for library programs and perhaps a handout of one of the yoga poses for the kids to take home to show their parents.

Advice

- Remember you are working with preschoolers; their attention spans are limited. Don't take it personally if they don't/can't/won't sit still/close their eyes/breathe deeply/stop talking. Modulate your voice to help them follow along—if you get quiet, they will get quiet; if you get loud and animated, they will pay attention, but don't stay that way too long, or they will lose interest—change the pitch, tone, and direction of your voice to head into a new direction. This is easy when following along with the picture books because in the yoga book you can use the voices of the animal characters and in the meditation book you can change your voice to match the moods discussed by the narrator.

- Don't be afraid to be silly to help engage them. But also, don't force or shame anyone into participating. Some of the more cautious/introverted students may hang back a bit and just observe—that's OK too. They will join in when they feel comfortable, or maybe try to do poses on their own when they get home.

- Thirty to forty-five minutes is a great length of time for a preschool program to run; any longer than that and you are pushing your limits for their attention spans and need for snacks and bathroom breaks!

◎ Program Model: Chair Yoga for Lifelong Health

This is a wonderful program to offer on-site at your library and is great for beginners or people with limited mobility, but it can also be taught to staff during training, or the routine can be modified and shortened to be used as a little "stretch break" during long meetings or during the workday. Off-site, it is wonderfully versatile and can be used in care homes for the elderly or disabled, in schools, in corporate settings, community centers, and even hospitals. I've shared it at knitting conventions and mental health clinics. I even once taught a modified version of this routine to an ostomy support group at

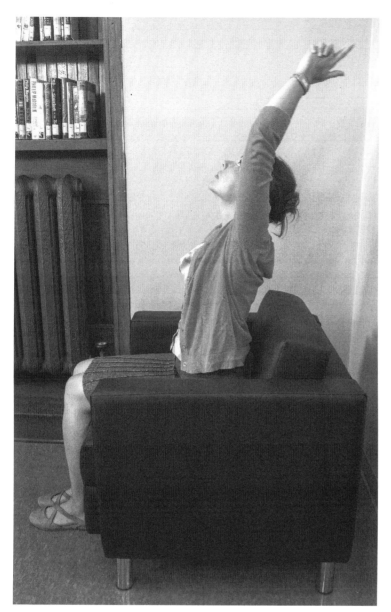

Figure 11.5. Chair Yoga is for all abilities.
Brendan Helmuth

the local hospital and they loved it! When doing outreach, think waaaaay outside the box here! But—and this is really important—only within the bounds of your training and comfort level.

Advanced Planning

Step 1. Pick what group or venue you'd like to approach, call them to explain what you are offering, and see if you can agree on a mutually beneficial date and time. Or, if doing this on-site, pick a time that works for your library's schedule. It's a great routine to add during a long day of training. The class should take about forty-five minutes to an hour, but can be shortened by doing fewer poses.

Step 2. Ask the group how much space they have available, how many people will be attending, and, if possible, glean the average mobility of the group and if there will be anyone in attendance you should plan to make modifications for. It's better to know ahead of time than to be surprised. Confirm the location has enough chairs (firm folding-style or desk chairs are ideal, but this can be done on couches or recliners too), and if not, plan to bring some, if possible. You may also want to bring blocks and mats. This program works well (with some modifications) for people in wheelchairs that have upper-body mobility.

Step 3. Check with your administration and the group to confirm you are covered for injury and/or liability in case you or someone in the class gets injured. It's always a good idea to print off liability waivers and have the students/patients and/or their caregivers sign ahead of time.

Step 4. Before the event, gather all the necessary materials (see "Materials Required" below).

Step 5. Look over the infographic (see pages 143–144) to familiarize yourself with the exercises and do a trial run with a staff member or volunteer ahead of time.

Step 6. If offering the program on-site at your library, be sure to advertise.

Materials Required

- Liability waivers, if using (if off-site, check with the location)
- Singing bowl or bell or gong
- Chairs
- Yoga mats (sometimes, if the students have difficulty with balance, or the floors are very slippery, I put mats under the chairs for extra grip)
- Blocks (sometimes used to place under the feet of shorter people who can't easily make contact with the floor)
- Evaluation forms, if using
- Yoga books and other materials from the library's collection to show what is available to borrow (and a pop-up library for checkouts if you have that service at your library)
- Yoga consent cards, if you plan on giving hands-on adjustments

Budget Details

$0. This program shouldn't cost you anything, except the transportation costs to get to the location (if going off-site), assuming you already have the singing bowl and (optional) mats/blocks, and chairs.

Day-of-Event

Step 1. Introduce yourself to the group and welcome everyone. Have everyone complete a liability waiver. Explain briefly what Chair Yoga is and see who has tried it (or regular yoga) before. Remind everyone to only do what feels good for their body and to not push beyond that.

Step 2. Have everyone sit comfortably on their chair, with their feet firmly planted on the ground and their hands in their laps, resting on their knees. If their feet can't reach the ground, place blocks under their feet for support. Start with some breath awareness.

Step 3. Follow along with the poses and instructions on the infographic (see pages 143–144).

Step 4. Bring everyone out of the final *Savasana* (which can be done in the chair or on the floor) by ringing the bell/singing bowl.

Chair Yoga

FOR LIFELONG HEALTH

Chair yoga can be done by people of all ages and abilities. This routine is a great way to stay active while seated at the office, in front of the TV, on an airplane, or at the library! Grab a friend for some relaxing partner-work.

www.jenncarson.com
www.yogainthelibrary.com
www.physicalliteracyinthelibrary.com

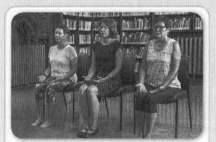

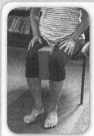

2. Block Between Knees Place a block between your knees and squeeze gently with your thighs. This will help engage your pelvic floor muscles. Take 5 deep belly breaths.

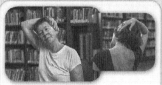

3. Neck Stretches Place your right hand over your head and onto your left ear. Gently pull your head to the right shoulder. Take 5 breaths. Repeat on the other side.

1. Proper Chair Posture Sit on the edge of your chair with your feet flat on the floor. If it is more comfortable, put a pillow behind your lower back or blocks under your feet. Roll your shoulders away from your ears and drop your breath into your belly. Inhale, belly goes out. Exhale, belly pulls in. Relax your jaw. Palms can roll up toward the ceiling or rest downward on your thighs.

5. Hand Stretches
(a) With arms out straight in front of you, point fingers toward the floor. (b) Raise fingers toward the ceiling. (c) Rotate fingers toward each other. (d) Rotate fingers away from each other. Repeat entire sequence 10 times.

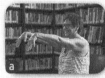
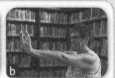

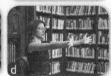

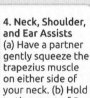

4. Neck, Shoulder, and Ear Assists
(a) Have a partner gently squeeze the trapezius muscle on either side of your neck. (b) Hold to the count of 5 and then release. Repeat 5 times. (c) Pull gently on the edges of the ears with the tips of the fingers, starting at the top of the ears and working down to the lobes. Switch and give your partner a turn.

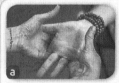
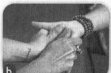
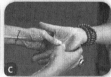

6. Hand Stretch Assists (a) Have a partner reach their pinky fingers in between your middle and index finger and your pinky and ring finger. (b) They will reach their fingers around the back of your hand and press their thumbs into the palm of your hand, (c) making gentle strokes toward your wrist and fingers. This releases the connective tissue in the hands. Massage for a few minutes and then switch hands. Then give your partner a hand massage.

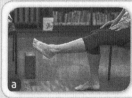
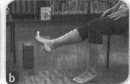

7. Foot Stretches (a) Lift one foot, point and flex foot 10 times. (b) Rotate ankle in clockwise circles 5 times, then counterclockwise 5 times. Lower foot and repeat on the other side.

Jenn Carson is a physical literacy expert, yoga instructor, librarian, and author of *Get Your Community Moving: Physical Literacy Programs for All Ages.*

Figure 11.6.

Chair Yoga for Lifelong Health

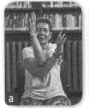 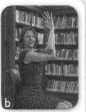

8. Eagle Arms (a) Raise bent elbows with palms facing each other. Swim right arm under the left arm. Hold for 5 breaths. Repeat on other side, swimming left arm under right arm. (b) Advanced version: bring palms to touch and lift elbows to 90°, so they are in line with your shoulders.

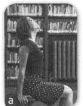 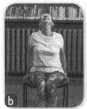

9. Seated Back Bend (a) Sit on the edge of your chair with feet planted on the floor. Place your hands next to your hips and push into the chair's surface (or grab the edge of the chair). (b) Lift chin and chest gently toward the ceiling. Take 5 deep belly breaths.

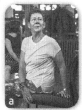 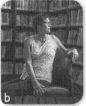

10. Seated Twist (a) Sit on the edge of your chair. Place your right hand on your left knee or on the outside left edge of the chair. Place your left hand on the seat behind you or, (b) if you have the shoulder mobility, on the back of the chair. Inhale and sit up tall. Exhale and look over your left shoulder. Take 5 deep breaths. Repeat on the other side.

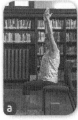 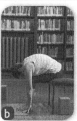 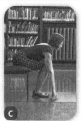 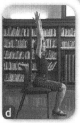

11. Seated Sun Salutation (a) Sit on the edge of your chair and inhale, lifting arms overheard. (b) Exhale, bend over and reach toward your toes. (c) Inhale, straighten your back and look up. Exhale, bend over and reach toward your toes again. (d) Inhale, reach your arms overhead. Exhale, bring your hands to your lap. Repeat entire sequence 5 times.

12. Twist Inhale and reach your hands toward the ceiling. Exhale and fold over your legs. Place both hands on the floor or on a block. Inhale, reach your right arm in the air, twisting your torso gently to the right. Exhale and lower arm. Repeat on the left side and then repeat both sides 5 times each.

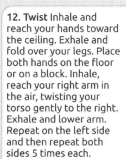 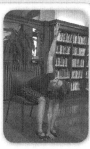

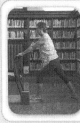

13. Warrior One with Chair Stand behind your chair (preferably with a mat under your feet). Holding on to the chair back, step your left leg back about 3 feet, positioning your left foot at a 45° and bend your right knee. Hold for 5 breaths. Repeat on the other side.

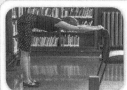

14. Down Dog Holding on to the back of the chair, walk your feet back and pivot at your waist until your back is parallel to the floor. Press down through your armpits and relax your jaw. Hold for 5 breaths. Come up slowly to prevent dizziness.

16. *Savasana* with Legs on Chair Lie on the floor with your lower legs resting on the chair. Spread the arms out to your sides with palms

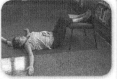

facing up. Relax your forehead and jaw. If you'd like, place a beanbag on your belly to help focus your breathing. Inhale, beanbag lifts toward the ceiling, exhale beanbag lowers down. Stay as long as you'd like. Come out slowly and mindfully.

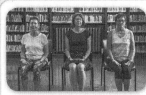

15. Meditation Come into proper seated position (pose #1) with your hands resting in your lap. Drop your breath down into your belly. Breathing in, belly goes away from the body. Breathing out, belly pulls in toward the back of the chair. Follow the breath in and out, counting 1 on the inhale and 2 on the exhale, then 3 on the inhale, 4 on the exhale. Go all the way to 10 and then start again. If your mind wanders off mid-count, start again at 1. Continue for at least 5-10 minutes.

Program design by Jenn Carson • Photography by Drew Gilbert • Layout by Brendan Helmuth

Figure 11.7.

Step 5. Thank everyone for coming and ask if anyone would like to share a bit about their experience during the class. Give out evaluation forms to participants to encourage them to share how they felt during the practice anonymously and to offer any advice for how to best suit their needs during the next session.

Step 6. If you brought along some items from your library's collection, share them with the group and let them know what yoga-related materials are available at your library. If your patrons can't leave the facility, this would be an excellent opportunity to offer to do a book deposit or register them for your books-by-mail service (if you have one).

Advice

- Based on the information supplied on the liability waivers, and perhaps what has been shared by their caregivers, make sure to modify the class to suit the needs of the students. If you feel like someone's complex health issues are more complicated than you are trained to handle, say as much. You are not a doctor. It isn't worth someone getting hurt over because your ego got in the way.
- Depending on the location of the class and ages of participants, you may wish to modify the length of time. The class is designed to be one hour, but with the elderly or infirm, twenty to thirty minutes of activity may be enough.
- Sometimes people who don't do a lot of physical activity can get easily discouraged and grumbly about it. Don't take it personally. Don't let it detract from the class, and offer everyone gentle encouragement.
- Remind everyone they can skip any posture that feels too difficult and come back to their belly breathing.

⊚ Program Model: Yoga for Heartache

Ahh, grief. Trauma and loss—and their emotional bedfellow grief—are inescapable parts of living. By the time you reach middling adulthood, you are almost guaranteed to have

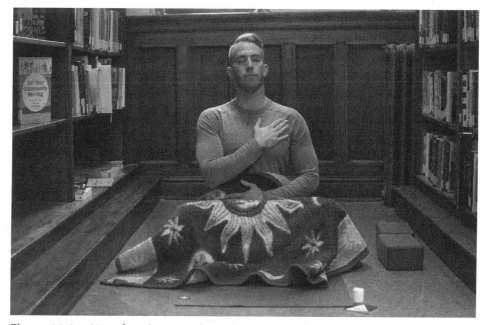

Figure 11.8. Yoga for when your heart hurts. *Ebony Scott*

YOGA FOR HEARTACHE

Grab a blanket, some blocks, and follow along with this quiet, reflective, restorative sequence to help heal your heart — no matter what caused its suffering.

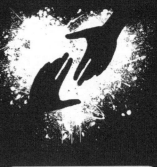

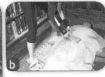

1. Belly Breathing (a) Lie on the back, covered with a blanket if preferred. (b) Place a bean bag on the belly. The feet roll out to the sides and the palms turn up to face the ceiling. Take a deep breath and feel the bean bag lift toward the ceiling, on the exhale feel the bean bag lower toward the spine. Repeat 5 times.

2. Easy Pose Sit in a crossed-legged position, with blocks under the knees for support. Option to place blanket around shoulders for comfort. Take 5 deep breaths.

3. Easy Twist From Easy Pose, place the left hand on the right knee and the right hand around the back with the palm facing outward. Take an inhale and on the exhale look over the right shoulder. Repeat, twisting to the left this time.

4. Lion's Breath From a kneeling position, curl the toes under. Rotate the palms 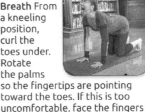 so the fingertips are pointing toward the toes. If this is too uncomfortable, face the fingers forward. Raise the chin toward the ceiling. Take a large inhale through the nostrils and exhale loudly through the mouth, sticking out the tongue. Take 3 normal breaths and repeat.

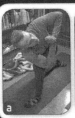

5. Cat/Cow (a) From a kneeling position, place both hands on the floor, shoulder-width apart. Place a block between the thighs and squeeze. Press through the palms. Inhale and look toward the ceiling. (b) Exhale and arch the back upward, tucking the chin. Repeat both poses 9 more times.

6. Crescent Moon From a kneeling position, step the right foot between the hands. Pressing in through the top of the left foot and the sole of the right foot, lift the hands toward the ceiling. If this is difficult for the shoulders, rest the hands on the bent right knee. Hold for 5 breaths. Repeat on the left side. Return to kneeling.

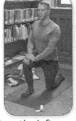

7. Crescent Lunge From a kneeling position, step the right foot between the hands. Curl the left toes under and lift the left knee off the ground. Bring the hands overhead, or to the right knee. Hold for 5 breaths. Repeat on the left side. Return to kneeling.

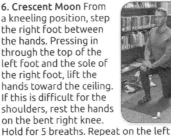

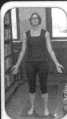

8. Twisted Crescent Lunge From a kneeling position, step the right foot between the hands. Curl the left toes under and lift the left knee off the ground. (a) Reach the left arm over the right knee, hooking the elbow and twisting toward the right. Bring hands to prayer position at heart center. Hold for 5 breaths. Repeat on left side. (b) For more of a challenge, lower the left hand toward the ground and reach the right arm toward the ceiling.

11. Halfmoon Pose (a) From a standing position, place a block on the highest edge in front of the right foot. Reach down with the right hand and hold on to the block. Lift the left leg in the air, the same height as the torso. Reach the left arm overhead and rotate the torso to the left. Hold for 5 breaths. Repeat on the left leg. (b) For more of a challenge, grasp the left foot in the left hand and arch the back.

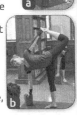

9. Mountain Pose From standing, lift the toes and lower them slowly, feeling the floor solid underfoot. Lift heart toward the ceiling. Relax the shoulders. Relax the jaw. Keep the pelvis neutral. Take 5 breaths.

10. Arm Swings From a standing position, plant the feet on the outer edges of the mat and bend the knees slightly. Start gently swinging the arms back and forth across the body. Slowly increase the speed, keeping the arms loose in their sockets. Keep the heels planted. Decrease the speed until coming to a stop in Mountain Pose.

Figure 11.9.

Yoga Consent Cards These double-sided paper cards are meant to be displayed next to the mat, so the teacher can tell if the student would like to be touched or not. The student can change their mind mid-way through class and simply flip their card over with no need to draw attention to themselves. This gives the student a sense of freedom and empowerment.

12. Lumberjack Swings (a) From a standing position, plant the feet on the outer edges of the mat and bend the knees, coming into a high squat. Clasp the hands together as if holding an ax. (b) Inhaling sharply through the nose, reach the arms over head. Keeping the arms overhead, exhale lightly. (c) Repeat inhale/exhale three more times but on the last exhale yell "ARGHHH!" while exhaling loudly through the mouth. (d) Bring the hands down between the feet as if chopping a large log. Repeat entire sequence 2 more times.

13. Standing Split (a) From a standing position, reach down and place both hands on the mat, bending the knees as needed. Walk the hands closer to the foot while lifting the right leg in

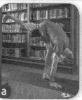

the air. If possible, hold the standing leg's ankle with one hand. Hold for 5 breaths. Repeat on the other side. (b) For more of a challenge, hold the standing leg's ankle with both hands and bring the chin toward the standing leg.

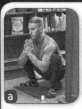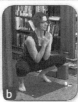

14. Yoga Squat (a) From a standing position, plant the feet on the outer edges of the mat and bend the knees, coming into a high squat. Place a block on the mat and sit on the block (on whatever height feels most comfortable). Bring the hands to prayer position at the chest and press the palms together. Take 5 breaths and return to standing. (b) For more of a challenge, remove the block and lower your hips toward the mat, keeping the heels planted.

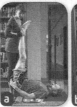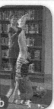

15. Shoulder Stand (a) Place a folded blanket across the middle of the mat and lie on the blanket with shoulders touching its edge, the head resting on the mat. Walk the feet in close to the sit bones and press into the feet, lifting the hips. Place a block underneath the sacrum in a comfortable position. Lift the legs in the air and bring the hands to the lower back, the elbows resting on the mat. Have a teacher or partner offer support for the legs, if preferred. Hold for 10 breaths. Do not look from side to side; keep the chin tucked. Lower the legs. (b) For a more challenging version, do not use a block and support the lumbar spine with the hands. Bring the elbows in as close to the spine as possible. Reach the balls of the feet toward the ceiling. Have a teacher or partner support the legs, if preferred.

16. Fish Pose (a) Lie on the mat and bring the soles of the feet together, the knees draping open to the sides. For added support place blocks under the knees. Reach the arms overhead, creating a halo shape. Hold for 5 breaths. (b) For a more challenging version, lie on the mat with the legs out long. Tuck the thumbs under the hips and press the elbows into the mat, lifting the chest toward the ceiling. Arch the back and rest the crown of the head on the mat, chin stretching away from the torso.

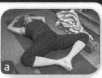

17. *Savasana* (a) Lie on the mat, covered with a blanket, if that feels comfortable. Place a bean bag on the belly. Roll the feet to the side and the palms toward the ceiling. (b) Consented teacher assists can include a gentle squeeze to the *Marma* points of the feet. (c) A gentle alignment of the neck vertebrae. (d) A gentle ear pull. (e) A gentle shoulder press. Close the eyes and continue with Belly Breathing for at least 5 minutes. The teacher rings the bell to bring everyone out.

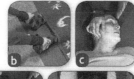
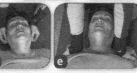

18. Heart Meditation Sit in Easy Pose, with blanket, if preferred. Place the right hand to the heart and

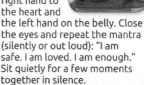

the left hand on the belly. Close the eyes and repeat the mantra (silently or out loud): "I am safe. I am loved. I am enough." Sit quietly for a few moments together in silence.

Program design by Jenn Carson • Photography by Ebony Scott • Layout by Brendan Helmuth

Figure 11.10.

experienced the death of a loved one (even if "only" a pet), been subjected to harassment or violence, or experienced an accident, natural disaster, or medical crisis. For some people, their resiliency seems to allow them to bounce back—or at least muddle through their days carrying some residual pain around with them—for others, grief is a tsunami they battle just to get out of bed in the morning. No matter your personal experience with trauma, offering a trauma-informed mindfulness-based yoga class at your library is an excellent way to support those in your community who may be suffering.[4] Which may, in fact, be most of us on any given day. I try to offer this program especially around the holidays, like Christmas or Valentine's Day, to give people a place to go to heal and where they don't have to put on a fake smile and suffer stoically through another round of "Joy to the World" while swallowing the lump in their throat. This class can be offered on-site at your own library to the general public or can be taken off-site to various community organizations, churches, funeral homes, hospitals, or recovery shelters.

Advance Planning

Step 1. Find an instructor with a background in trauma-informed yoga teaching or, if you are a yoga teacher yourself, following along with the sequence starting on page 146, pay close attention to the special instructions. This isn't a regular yoga class; extra care is needed when people are in pain. Read the "Advice" section carefully for more tips on how to prepare and deliver this class.

Step 2. Pick a day and time for the program and book the room. I try to offer the class near triggering holidays for those experiencing loss, such as Christmas, Memorial Day (Remembrance Day in Canada), or Valentine's Day, or in correspondence with days of awareness that affect those groups who have traditionally experienced emotional and physical abuse, such as Sisters in Spirit Week (to honor missing and murdered indigenous women) or Transgender Awareness Week. Good class times are often in the evening, when people can feel most alone after the busyness of the workday has passed, but I've also taught this program on weekend mornings and afternoons with much success. A room where you can black out the windows and have minimal atmospheric noise is preferred though not essential. If you are teaching the program off-site, make sure the room meets these goals.

Step 3. Decide if this is going to be a drop-in or pre-registration-required event and how many you can serve. Make a sign-up sheet, if required.

Step 4. Create liability waivers. Don't even think about taking photos. Create evaluation forms, if using.

Step 5. Print consent cards. They are available for free download from http://www .jenncarson.com/assets/yoga_consent_card.pdf.

Step 6. Gather all materials required for the program (see below for a list) and secure funding if needed.

Step 7. Advertise your event, if open to the general public and not being provided for a specific group. Make an eye-catching poster. Share on social media. Consider making a promo video for YouTube or Facebook Live. Add to your print or digital calendar. Most importantly, share with community groups that may best be able to reach your desired audience: halfway houses and women's shelters, veterans' organizations, PTSD and addiction treatment clinics, therapy and recovery organizations, doctors' offices, local chapters of Alcoholics Anonymous, Narcotics Anonymous, and Al-Anon. Share with local churches, fellowships, and funeral homes. Grief is everywhere.

Materials Required

- Yoga mats and blocks
- Consent cards
- Liability waivers
- Evaluation forms, if using
- Flameless candles or lamps for soft lighting
- Singing bell or bowl
- Beanbags
- Blankets

Budget Details

$0–$500+. Depending on whether you already have the props available to host a yoga class, this could be an incredibly cheap production or require a serious investment. If you are hiring a teacher, ask if the teacher can provide the items you don't have. Look for community wellness or recovery grants to cover the cost of the materials.

Day of Event

Step 1. If you are preparing to teach the class, ground yourself at least ten minutes before the beginning of the program. In order to teach a trauma-informed class you need to settle any stress or distracting elements you may be carrying within yourself and put them into a safe emotional container for the duration of the class.

Step 2. Prepare the room for your students' arrival. Shade the windows so that other patrons or passerby cannot see in, dim the lights, and use flameless candles (I like the little LED tea lights) and low-wattage lamps. The room should feel like a safe, cozy, welcoming space. Put out the mats, props, and blankets so that the students only have to come in and choose a spot. Have the liability waivers and consent cards handy.

Step 3. Greet your students and have them complete the waiver. Encourage them to choose a mat and thank them for coming.

Step 4. Once everyone has arrived, let them know where the exits and bathrooms are. Explain that there will be optional touch adjustments during the class. Hand out the consent cards and explain how they can put the cards next to their mats to let you know whether they would like an adjustment. Assure them that they can change their mind at any point in the class by flipping their cards over. Since the cards are the same color on both sides, no one can tell what anyone else's card says. Clarify that it is perfectly normal to either want or not want to be touched and that you will in no way be offended or take it personally, that this is *their* choice and the power rests with them to decide how they feel in any given moment and you promise to respect that.

Step 5. Assure them that if at any point during the class they feel triggered, uncomfortable, or simply don't want to do a pose, they can return to their mat and rest in any easy sitting pose or Child's Pose. Demonstrate to show them their options.

Step 6. Following along with the infographic on pages 146–147 and lead students through the sequence provided.

Step 7. Bring the class to a close and thank everyone for coming. Keep the room as quiet and dim as possible while still allowing for socializing. Don't rush anyone to leave. Distribute evaluation forms, if using.

Step 8. Clean up the room. Record stats. Exhale.

- As yoga and meditation teachers, we are in the habit of having students focus on their breath. During stressful situations or while emotionally triggered, focusing on the breath (which can lead to focusing on the chest and heart rate) can actually be more upsetting for the student. They may be able to feel their heart racing or their breath becoming quick and shallow, or feel like they can't get enough of it, and this may produce panic. In these situations, it is best to remind students to focus on something more grounding and unchanging, such as feeling their feet planted on the ground (if they are sitting in a chair or standing) or making a soft fist with their hands and feeling the pressure of their fingers and then gently releasing their grip. Once students have more experience with yoga and meditation, the breath can be used more skillfully in times of duress, but it isn't an appropriate focus point during a public class of trauma-informed yoga with students who may be strangers to you and whose practice history is unknown. In this case it is best to remind students at different points during the class that if they are experiencing emotional discomfort, to focus on their feet planted on the mat or their hands on their thighs (or wherever these body parts are at the moment you say it).
- I like to assure students at any point in time, if they feel uncomfortable (or need a bathroom break), they have permission to leave the class. I only ask that they give me the "thumbs-up" sign on the way out. I tell them that if they don't give me the thumbs-up, I'm going to assume they are emotionally upset or have an injury and I (or my assistant) will follow them to make sure they are OK. If you can have an assistant available as an emotional support person during class, this can be their job, as well as to help with adjustments or the placement of props.
- Some trauma-informed yoga instructors prefer not to touch students at all, as they feel this could be potentially triggering. I follow the TIMBo (Trauma Informed Mind Body) school of thought that says offering non-confrontational, consensual, safe touch is an opportunity for healing and empowerment.[5] You do what feels right for you.
- Resist the urge to play music during the class, unless you really need some soothing ambient tunes to drown out the background noise in your facility. If so, choose only instrumental. Music can be very distracting to students, and depending on the grief they are experiencing, potentially upsetting (e.g., hearing a love song during a period of loss of a spouse or partner).

SUGGESTIONS FOR CIRCULATING COLLECTION

Airplane Yoga: Your Emergency Safety Manual for Relieving In-Flight Stress by Rachel Lehmann-Haupt and Bess Abrahams.
New York: Riverhead, 2003. ISBN 978-1-57322-352-2; Paperback; US$13.00/Can$19.50.

While this older title may not be something you add to your collection, if you already have a copy or can snag one through ILL, it's a great foundation for building a program called Yoga for Frequent Flyers or Travel Wellness (for more a generalized audience). While this may not be a big draw in a rural farming area with a small population where people don't travel a lot (but hey—even the Amish have to sit for long distances in their buggies!), it would definitely be popular in a big-city public library branch or may appeal in an academic library where people commute on the train regularly. Create a little handout tip sheet they can tuck into their purse or carry-on to remind them of the routine during their trip. Here are some highlights found in the book: "Heavy Luggage Wrist Rolls," "Long Line Leg Reviver," "Meal Tray Meditation," "Nosy Neighbor Chest Opener," and "Barf Bag Wrist Relief." If nothing else, reading this manual will give you and your staff a good giggle. Bonus points if you can convince your administration to let you run the program as outreach at your local airport or train/bus station.

Asanas for Autism and Special Needs: Yoga to Help Children with their Emotions, Self-Regulation and Body Awareness by Shawnee Thornton Hardy.
London: Jessica Kingsley, 2015. ISBN 978-1-84905-988-6; Paperback; US$19.95/Can$19.95.

This is an excellent book to have on your shelves for parents, teachers, and anyone else who works with children with special needs. It identifies how yoga and meditation can help those with ADD/ADHD, ASD, Fragile X syndrome, Down syndrome, and Prader-Willi syndrome. There are some useful activities in here for promoting body awareness (including directional awareness) and acceptance. There are pictures to illustrate each pose, a structured and consistent layout for instruction, and a clear, methodical delivery that readers will surely appreciate. Highly recommended for circulating and professional collection.

Chair Yoga: Sit, Stretch, and Strengthen Your Way to a Happier, Healthier You by Kristin McGee.
New York: William Morrow, 2017. ISBN 978-0-0624-8644-8; Paperback; US$18.99.

Believe it or not, there aren't many Chair Yoga books on the market (there are a few DVDs). This one, from celebrity trainer Kristin McGee, is peppy and bright with lots of clear instructional photos patrons can use to practice at home and work. Older audiences might have a hard time relating to all the young, blond, California-fit-ness jumping off the pages, but the methodology is solid and I would feel confident recommending it.

Mindfulness Skills for Trauma and PTSD: Practices for Recovery and Resilience by Rachel Goldsmith Turow.
New York: W.W. Norton, 2017. ISBN 978-0-393-77126-4; Paperback; US$27.95/Can$36.95.

An excellent reference to have on hand to recommend to patrons looking for alternative ways to deal with trauma and PTSD-related issues, including complex trauma systems. Also excellent to flip through if you are teaching a Yoga for Heartache program (see page 145 for program model) and need some tips for how to deal with certain aspects of the students' experiences or some useful teaching tools,

(continued)

such as the "Boats on a River" exercise on page 75, or "Spot the Success" exercise on page 110. Even those not suffering from the above-mentioned issues can benefit from this work. The author is also realistic about managing the expectations of her readers with gentle reminders that "mindfulness practice cannot solve all problems" and needs to be combined with other positive actions. Highly recommended for your circulating collection and also as a teaching tool for anyone working with victims of trauma.

Overcoming Trauma through Yoga: Reclaiming Your Body by David Emerson and Elizabeth Hopper.
Berkeley, CA: North Atlantic Books, 2011. ISBN 978-1-55643-969-8; Paperback; US$19.95/Can$22.95.

Whether or not you feel comfortable offering trauma-recovery yoga programs in your library, this is an important read for anyone teaching yoga to the general population since most people have experienced trauma at some point in their lives, either directly or as witnesses. In this book, the authors share how in the US alone, 7.7 million adults suffer from PTSD and domestic violence is the leading cause of injury to women aged fifteen to forty-four, more common than car accidents, muggings, and cancer combined. This means the majority of people entering your library on any given day are suffering, most often in silence. Trauma creates a destructive feedback loop of negative self-talk, obsessive hyper-vigilance, and uncontrolled rage or disassociation in the body. The goal of yoga is to get people back in touch with the bodies they have known as shaming, uncontrollable, or broken, and help them to accept reality. Teachers can create safe spaces for them in the library by offering yoga programs that follow the important rules listed in this book, such as not using visualizations, minimizing commands and using inviting language instead, offering verbal and visual assists instead of physical ones, and keeping the noise and light level consistent. Includes sample classes and at-home exercises for trauma recovery accompanied by photos, making it an excellent addition to the circulating and/or professional development collections.[6]

Yoga for Children with Autism Spectrum Disorders: A Step-by-Step Guide for Parents and Caregivers by Dion E. Betts and Stacey W. Betts.
London: Jessica Kingsley, 2006. ISBN 978-1-84310-817-7; Paperback; US$18.95.

This thoughtful manual is written by a husband (an educator) and wife (an attorney) team who have an autistic son, Joshua, as well as four other children. Joshua has written an introduction to the book explaining that while he thinks "yoga is weird," he has actually learned how to enjoy the sensation of having his head upside down and found that focusing on his breath relieved his stress and helped him self-stim less (a stereotypical example of stimming would be hand flapping when bored or anxious). The book has an excellent introduction explaining many of the symptoms children on the autism spectrum display and how yoga can help, making this an excellent reference for parents, teachers, and also for library staff members who may encounter patrons with ASD in their programs. As the Bettses point out on pages 18–20, yoga increases muscle tone and stamina, helps alleviate gross and fine motor delay and weight gain, improves balance, quiets an overloaded nervous system, and helps people accept themselves, even with their challenges. This is an excellent step-by-step guide to the more accessible *Asanas* complete with detailed instructions, pictures, emotional impact, and modifications for people on the spectrum. The book ends with suggested short practice sequences and a comprehensive introduction to five different breathing exercises (*Pranayama*) complete with photos and helpful hints. Written from a place of love, respect, and deep understanding, it is a must-have resource for any public or school library collection.[7]

Yoga for Pregnancy and Birth: Improve Your Wellbeing throughout Pregnancy and Beyond by Uma Dinsmore-Tula.
London: Hodder Education, 2008. ISBN 978-1-444-10097-6; Paperback; US$16.99.

The nice thing about this book is that there is a free audio version available at library.teachyourself.com. The material is comprehensive and text heavy with line-drawn illustrations, and it will appeal to the mother-to-be who likes to research every last detail, the advanced yogi, or those who are wishing to teach yoga to pregnant patrons and want as much information as possible. For the beginner practitioner or someone looking for a quick reference guide, I would recommend *Yoga for Pregnancy, Birth, and Beyond* by Françoise Barbira Freedman (DK, 2004), and for the more spiritual-sided mama-to-be, I'd recommend *Bountiful, Beautiful, Blissful: Experience the Natural Power of Pregnancy and Birth with Kundalini Yoga and Meditation* by Gurmukh Kaur Khalsa (St. Martin's Griffin, 2004) which was my favorite during pregnancy. Remember to seek out a teacher with special training for teaching a Yoga for Pregnancy class at your library, as there are special safety considerations that need to be taken into consideration. If pregnant women come to your regular class, make sure you feel comfortable modifying the poses for them and that they understand the risks.

SUGGESTIONS FOR PROFESSIONAL DEVELOPMENT COLLECTION

101 Mindful Arts-Based Activities to Get Children and Adolescents Talking: Working with Severe Trauma, Abuse and Neglect Using Found and Everyday Objects by Dawn D'Amico.
Philadelphia: Jessica Kingsley, 2017. ISBN 978-1-78592-731-7; Paperback; US$24.95.

Before the title throws you off, don't worry that anyone is expecting you to be an artist, therapist, or social worker (though librarians do become de facto versions at times). I recommend this book because there are some extremely useful exercises that can be included during mindfulness programs for teens and children, especially helpful when doing outreach at juvenile detention centers, homeless shelters, occupational therapy clinics, multicultural/immigration centers, hospitals, or any

(continued)

other locations where your young patrons may have been under stress. A bonus is the lesson plans are low cost since they use primarily found and recycled materials. The activities are divided into either visual, verbal, or tactile categories and geared toward kids aged five to seventeen. Some may be too "therapy-like" for a library program, but there are some real gems in here that promote mindfulness and literacy, such as "Life Story Book" (creating an oral or written history of positive memories and helpers in the student's life), "I Love Being Me" (balloons of words or drawings of positive things the students experience about themselves), "When I Was Young" (blowing bubbles as a storytelling device), "Tornado" (creating water bottle tornadoes to talk about swirling thoughts, mixed emotions, or chaotic life events), "Open and Closed" (using curled and uncurled palms or entire bodies to talk about open and closed feelings), and many more.

Mindful Work: How Meditation Is Changing Business from the Inside Out by David Gelles.
New York: First Mariner, 2016. ISBN 978-0-544-70525-8; Paperback; US$14.95.

Are your staff or administration still not sold on the idea that adding meditation breaks to the workday or sending staff for mindfulness training is a worthy investment? Place this book (or the audiobook version) in their hands (preferably accompanied with a nice cup of tea and *zazen* cushion) and see if they don't change their minds after reading it.

Yoga for Grief Relief: Simple Practices for Transforming Your Grieving Mind & Body by Antonio Sausys.
Oakland, CA: New Harbinger, 2014. ISBN 978-1-60882-818-0; Paperback; US$21.95.

This helpful book works from the premise that most of us are walking around in a state of unacknowledged grief, carrying invisible traumas and sorrows (small and large) that our society deems unacceptable to express but that cannot go away without processing. It suggests that while talk therapy is important, we also need to take a body-centric approach to dealing with reality and the inevitability of suffering in our lives. I really like how the book goes into multiple aspects of grief, not just how it affects you physically and emotionally, but also mentally (such as experiencing absentmindedness), socially (such as withdrawing), spiritually (such as feeling angry at God), and behaviorally (such as assuming mannerisms of the deceased). Using breathing techniques, relaxation exercises, meditation, and very simple but incredibly effective movements, such as "elbow bending," this manual is devoid of what we have come to think of as "traditional" yoga poses (there's not a Down Dog in sight!). In reality, this book is very much grounded in the tenets of yoga as a spiritually nourishing and physically healing practice, which is what one would hope from a book addressing those in the throes of grief. Highly recommended for your circulating collection but also for anyone teaching students who are experiencing recovery from trauma (which, on some level, is most of us). Especially good to read if you are planning to teach Yoga for Heartache (page 145).

Yoga Therapy for Children with Autism and Special Needs by Louise Goldberg. New York: W. W. Norton, 2013. ISBN 978-0-393-70785-4; Hardcover; US$24.95/ Can$29.95.

Like Goldberg, I also began my yoga teaching career working with kids with emotional-behavioral disorders, low- or high-functioning autism, learning disabilities, or other emotional or neurological issues that affect their daily lives. I wish I had had this textbook when I began teaching. While this book primarily focuses on yoga *therapy*—which is the application of yoga techniques for specific conditions— it is a useful read for any yoga teacher working with children in school or public libraries, as many have these issues (diagnosed or otherwise). It discusses the benefits of yoga, meditation, and relaxation breathing for children with specific special needs, such as physical disabilities, emotional-behavioral disorders, autism spectrum disorders, ADHD, and sensory processing disorder. There are many helpful photo examples of hands-on modifications. And (how wonderful!) it includes games for language development, spatial awareness, and empathy (follow the leader/mirror neuron games). Read this book.

🌀 Key Points

- Outreach programs can bring yoga and meditation to marginalized populations in your community who can't make it to the library for a variety of reasons, or who aren't aware these programs exist.
- Outreach programs can create new library users and increase circulation and program statistics.
- Outreach can be both online and in person and is only limited by budget and imagination.
- Inreach programs can bring yoga and meditation to library staff who are often suffering from work-related stress.
- When working with students with exceptionalities or under special circumstances, it is important to modify the program to meet their needs. The same rules apply whether we are offering the program on-site or in the community.
- Many existing yoga and meditation programs designed for delivery in the library can be modified for outreach. Likewise, many outreach programs designed for specific populations can also be offered on-site, or to staff during training.
- Collection development of yoga and meditation materials for special populations is important, and there are many books on the market available for both the general public and as resources for professional use.

🌀 Notes

1. Kelly Starrett, Juliet Starrett, and Glen Cordoza, *Deskbound: Standing Up to a Sitting World* (Las Vegas: Victory Belt, 2016).
2. Louise Goldberg, *Yoga Therapy for Children with Autism and Special Needs* (New York: Norton, 2013).

3. Przemyslaw Wechterowicz and Emilia Dziubak, *Hug Me, Please!* (Lake Forest, CA: words & pictures, 2017).

4. Julia Dellitt, "This Nonprofit Organization Is Using Yoga to Help People Heal after Domestic Abuse," *Self*, May 21, 2018, https://www.self.com/story/nonprofit-organization-tough-as-milk-yoga-heal-after-domestic-abuse.

5. Suzanne E. Jones, "Mindful Touch: A Guide to Hands-On Support in Trauma-Sensitive Yoga," Yoga Service Council, 2018.

6. A different version of this book review first appeared on www.yogainthelibrary.com.

7. A different version of this book review first appeared on www.yogainthelibrary.com.

Bibliography

Aesop. "The Boy Who Cried Wolf." 1867 version. Lit2Go. Accessed November 16, 2018. http://etc.usf.edu/lit2go/35/aesops-fables/375/the-boy-who-cried-wolf/.

American Library Association (ALA). *Every Child Ready to Read @ Your Library*. Accessed November 10, 2018. http://everychildreadytoread.org/.

———. "Non-traditional Circulating Materials." Public Library Association. Accessed November 12, 2018. http://www.ala.org/pla/resources/tools/circulation-technical-services/nontraditional-circulating-materials.

American Osteopathic Association. "Maintaining a Regular Yoga Practice Can Provide Physical and Mental Health Benefits." *The Benefits of Yoga*. Accessed November 13, 2018. https://osteopathic.org/what-is-osteopathic-medicine/benefits-of-yoga/.

American Psychological Association. *Stress in America: The State of our Nation*. November 1, 2017. https://www.apa.org/news/press/releases/stress/2017/state-nation.pdf.

Biegel, Gina M. *Be Mindful & Stress Less*. Boulder, CO: Shambhala, 2018.

Block, Peter. *The Answer to How Is Yes: Acting on What Matters*. San Francisco: Berrett-Koehler, 2001.

Carson, Jenn. *Get Your Community Moving: Physical Literacy Programs for All Ages*. Chicago: ALA Editions, 2018.

———. *Physical Literacy: Movement-Based Programs in Libraries*. Survey. September 8, 2017. Personal author notes.

Centre for Koru Mindfulness. "About." Centre for Koru Mindfulness. Accessed November 10, 2018. https://korumindfulness.org/.

Chah, Ajahn. "Advice for Someone Who Is Dying." *Lion's Roar*, October 26, 2018. https://www.lionsroar.com/our-real-home-death/.

Chilton Pearce, Joseph. *Magical Child*. New York: Plume, 1992.

Christian, Linda A. "A Passion Deficit: Occupational Burnout and the New Librarian: A Recommendation Report." *Southeastern Librarian* 62, no. 4, article 2 (2016). https://digitalcommons.kennesaw.edu/seln/vol62/iss4/2.

Clarke, Tainya C., and Lindsey I. Black, Barbara J. Stussman, Patricia M. Barnes, and Richard L. Nahin. "Trends in the Use of Complementary Health Approaches among Adults: United States, 2002–2012." *National Health Statistics Reports*, no 79. Hyattsville, MD: National Center for Health Statistics, 2015. https://nccih.nih.gov/research/statistics/NHIS/2012.

Cronin, Doreen. "*Wiggle, Bounce, Stretch*." DoreenCronin.com. Accessed November 16, 2018. http://doreencronin.com/books/wiggle/.

Dellitt, Julia. "This Nonprofit Organization Is Using Yoga to Help People Heal after Domestic Abuse." *Self*, May 21, 2018. https://www.self.com/story/nonprofit-organization-tough-as-milk-yoga-heal-after-domestic-abuse.

Dudman, Jane. "Books Are the Best Medicine: How Libraries Boost Our Wellbeing." *Guardian*, October 10, 2018, https://www.theguardian.com/society/2018/oct/10/books-best-medicine-how-libraries-boost-wellbeing.

Dung, Phap. Introduction to *Making Space: Creating a Home Meditation Practice*, by Thich Nhat Hanh, 7–12. Berkeley, CA: Parallax, 2001.

Fairgray, Richard, and Jim Kraft. *Open in Case of Emergency*. New York: Sky Pony, 2017.

Fulweiler, Bernadette, and Rita Marie John. "Mind & Body Practices in the Treatment of Adolescent Anxiety." *Nurse Practitioner* 43, no. 8 (August 2018): 36–43.

Give Back Yoga Foundation. "Grant Information." Give Back Yoga Foundation. Accessed November 14, 2018. https://givebackyoga.org/about-our-non-profit-yoga-organization/grant-information/.

Goldberg, Louise. *Yoga Therapy for Children with Autism and Special Needs*. New York: Norton, 2013.

Government of Canada. "Canada's Law on Spam and Other Electronic Threats." Canada's Anti-Spam Legislation. 2017. http://fightspam.gc.ca/eic/site/030.nsf/eng/home.

Government of New Brunswick. "Appendix A: Standard Photo Release Form." *The New Brunswick Public Library Service Policy 1017*. January 2018. https://www2.gnb.ca/content/dam/gnb/Departments/nbpl-sbpnb/pdf/politiques-policies/1017_UseOfPhotos_Appendix.pdf.

———. "Appendix B: Sample Program Evaluation Form." *The New Brunswick Public Library Service Policy 1085*. July 2017. http://www2.gnb.ca/content/dam/gnb/Departments/nbpl-sbpnb/pdf/politiques-policies/1085_library-programs_appendix-b.pdf.

Hagell, Ann, Rakhee Shah, Russell Viner, Dougal Hargreaves, Laura Varnes, and Michelle Heys. "The Social Determinants of Young People's Health." *Health Foundation*, June 2018. https://www.health.org.uk/publication/social-determinants-young-peoples-health.

Hannaford, Carla. *Playing in the Unified Field: Raising & Becoming Conscious, Creative Human Beings*. Salt Lake City, UT: Great River Books, 2010.

Hanscom, Angela J. *Balanced and Barefoot: How Unrestricted Outdoor Play Makes for Strong, Confident, and Capable Children*. Oakland, CA: New Harbinger, 2016.

Harris, Dan. *10% Happier: How I Tamed the Voice in My Head, Reduced Stress without Losing My Edge, and Found Self-Help That Actually Works—A True Story*. New York: Dey Street Books, 2014.

Hartman, Bob, and Tim Raglin. *The Wolf Who Cried Boy*. London: Puffin, 2004.

Holton, Elizabeth. "People Visited Public Libraries More Than a Billion Times in 2015." Institute of Museum and Library Services. August 2, 2018. https://www.imls.gov/news-events/news-releases/people-visited-public-libraries-more-billion-times-2015.

Jails to Jobs. "How Practicing Meditation in Prison Can Help Inmates Cope." *Jails to Jobs* (blog). January 12, 2017. https://www.jailstojobs.org/how-practicing-meditation-in-prison-can-help-inmates-cope/.

Jones, Suzanne E. "Mindful Touch: A Guide to Hands-On Support in Trauma-Sensitive Yoga." Yoga Service Council. 2018.

Juhan, Deane. *Job's Body: A Handbook for Bodywork*. Barrytown, NY: Station Hill, 2003.

Kagan, Oleg. "Slow Info: Where Libraries, Reading, and Well-Being Converge." *EveryLibrary* (blog). January 23, 2018. https://medium.com/everylibrary/slow-info-where-libraries-reading-and-well-being-converge-44de619df0b8.

Katt, Ben. "The Art of Being Inefficient." *On Being Blog*. April 9, 2018. https://onbeing.org/blog/ben-katt-the-art-of-being-inefficient/.

Labyrinth Company. "Poly Canvas Mats." Labyrinth Company. Accessed November 10, 2018. https://www.labyrinthcompany.com/collections/poly-canvas-mats.

Lackner McLennan Insurance LTD. "Yoga Liability Insurance." Yoga Liability Insurance. Accessed November 15, 2018. https://www.yogainsurance.ca/.

Lamott, Anne. "12 Truths I Learned from Life and Writing." tinyTED. Accessed November 16, 2018. https://en.tiny.ted.com/talks/anne_lamott_12_truths_i_learned_from_life_and_writing.

Lee, Cyndi. "How to Practice Embodied Mindfulness." *Lion's Roar*, April 28, 2017. https://www.lionsroar.com/how-to-practice-embodied-mindfulness/?utm_content=bufferdda4b&utm_medium=social&utm_source=facebook.com&utm_campaign=buffer.

Lenstra, Noah. "Let's Move in Libraries." Let's Move in Libraries. 2017. http://www.LetsMoveLibraries.org/.

———. "Movement-Based Programs in U.S. and Canadian Public Libraries: Evidence of Impacts from an Exploratory Survey." *Evidence Based Library and Information Practice* 12, no. 4 (2017): 214–32.

Let's Move in Libraries. "Safety First." Let's Move in Libraries Resources. Accessed November 15, 2018. http://letsmovelibraries.org/resources/.

Lyons, Thomas, and William Dustin Cantrell. "Prison Meditation Movements and Mass Incarceration." *International Journal of Offender Therapy and Comparative Criminology* 60, no. 12 (2016): 1363–75. https://www.ncbi.nlm.nih.gov/pmc/articles/PMC4633398/.

MacMillan, Amanda. "It's Official: Yoga Helps Depression." *Time*, March 8, 2017. http://time.com/4695558/yoga-breathing-depression/.

———. "Yoga May Be Good for Stubborn Back Pain." *Time*, January 12, 2017. http://time.com/4632204/yoga-lower-back-pain/?iid=sr-link6.

Mazumdar, Anandashankar. "The Bikram Lawsuits and Why It Matters to You." Yoga Alliance. April 18, 2013. https://www.yogaalliance.org/Learn/Articles/bikram_lawsuits_4_18_2013.

McCrary, Meagan. *Pick Your Yoga Practice: Exploring and Understanding Different Styles of Yoga*. San Francisco: New World Library, 2013.

Moniz, Richard, Jo Henry, Joe Eshleman, Lisa Moniz, and Howard Slutzky. *Mindfulness Survey*. 2016. Private email correspondence with Richard Moniz, July 12, 2018.

Moore, Thomas. *The Re-enchantment of Everyday Life*. New York: Harper Perennial, 1997.

Nash-Degagne, Arielle. "Prenatal Yoga: The Essential Guidelines for Practice." Love Yoga Anatomy. Accessed November 16, 2018. https://loveyogaanatomy.com/prenatal-yoga-the-essential-guidelines-for-practice/.

Nhat Hanh, Thich. *Making Space: Creating a Home Meditation Practice*. Berkeley, CA: Parallax, 2001.

Online Computer Library Center (OCLC). *How Canadian Public Libraries Stack Up*. Online Computer Library Center. 2012. https://www.oclc.org/content/dam/oclc/reports/canadastackup/214109cef_how_libraries_stack_up.pdf.

Papageorge, Tiffany, and Erwin Madrid. *My Yellow Balloon*. San Francisco: Minoan Moon, 2014.

Pizer, Ann. "Downdog on the Go in Airports with Yoga Rooms." VeryWellFit. June 14, 2018. https://www.verywellfit.com/airport-yoga-rooms-3566838.

Prison Mindfulness Institute. "Books behind Bars." Prison Mindfulness Institute. Accessed November 1, 2018. https://www.prisonmindfulness.org/projects/books-behind-bars/.

Rinzler, Lordo. "10 Blunt Truths about Becoming a Meditation Teacher." *Elephant Journal*, July 21, 2015. https://www.elephantjournal.com/2015/07/10-blunt-truths-about-becoming-a-meditation-teacher/.

Rosen Schwartz, Corey, and Dan Santat. *Ninja Red Riding Hood*. New York: Scholastic, 2015.

Saad, Lydia. "Eight in 10 Americans Afflicted by Stress." Gallup. December 20, 2017. https://news.gallup.com/poll/224336/eight-americans-afflicted-stress.aspx.

Santat, Dan. *After the Fall: How Humpty Dumpty Got Back Up Again*. New York: Roaring Brook, 2017.

Shared Intelligence. *Library Rhyme Times and Maternal Mental Health—Action Research*. Accessed November 16, 2018. https://sharedintelligence.net/our-work-2-2/library-rhyme-times-and-maternal-mental-health-action-research/.

Smalley, Susan L., and Diana Winston. *Fully Present: The Science, Art, and Practice of Mindfulness*. New York: Da Capo Lifelong Books, 2010.

Solis, Sydney, and Melanie Sumner. *The Treasure in Your Heart: Stories and Yoga for Peaceful Children*. Boulder, CO: Mythic Yoga Studio, 2007.

Solis, Sydney, and Michele Trapani. *Storytime Yoga: Teaching Yoga to Children through Story*. Boulder, CO: Mythic Yoga Studio, 2006.

Starrett, Kelly, Juliet Starrett, and Glen Cordoza. *Deskbound: Standing Up to a Sitting World*. Las Vegas: Victory Belt, 2016.

Stephens, Mark. *Yoga Adjustments: Philosophy, Principles, and Techniques*. Berkeley, CA: North Atlantic Books, 2014.

Stixrud, William, and Ned Johnson. *The Self-Driven Child: The Science and Sense of Giving Your Kids More Control over Their Lives*. New York: Viking, 2018.

Stressed Teens. "Stress and Mindfulness." Stressed Teens: Resources. Accessed November 16, 2018. https://www.stressedteens.com/.

Suzuki, Shunryu. *Zen Mind, Beginner's Mind: Informal Talks on Zen Meditation and Practice*. Boulder, CO: Shambhala, 2011.

Therrien, Alex. "Lack of Exercise Puts One in Four People at Risk, WHO Says." BBC News. September 5, 2018. https://www.bbc.com/news/health-45408017.

Thomas, Naomi. "Yoga and Meditation on the Rise among US Adults and Kids." CNN. November 8, 2018. https://www.cnn.com/2018/11/08/health/yoga-meditation-rising-cdc-report/index.html?fbclid=IwAR16A8c5ax0Lr4eL8qeWpcm4R04hGDIg7s1M5FFRnN4zAw4Pv93ZNZke-TQ.

University of Toronto Libraries. "iRelax." Inforum Library. Accessed November 9, 2018. https://inforum.library.utoronto.ca/spaces/iRelax.

Vos, Aat. *3rd 4 All: How to Create a Relevant Public Space*. Rotterdam, Netherlands: nai010, 2017.

Wachter, Ronnie. "A Space Apart: College Libraries Contemplate Meditation Rooms." *American Libraries Magazine*, January 2, 2018. https://americanlibrariesmagazine.org/2018/01/02/library-meditation-rooms-space-apart/.

Wechterowicz, Przemyslaw, and Emilia Dziubak. *Hug Me, Please!* Lake Forest, CA: words & pictures, 2017.

Yoga Alliance. "Alliant Insurance." Yoga Alliance. Accessed November 10, 2018. https://www.yogaalliance.org/AlliantInsurance.

Index

About the Author

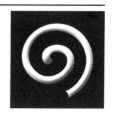

Jenn Carson is an internationally recognized expert in physical literacy, a professional yoga teacher, and the director of the L. P. Fisher Public Library in Woodstock, New Brunswick, Canada. She is the author of *Get Your Community Moving: Physical Literacy Programs for All Ages* (2018). She also blogs about her physical literacy adventures for Programming Librarian (www.programminglibrarian.org). You can find out more about her programs and research at www.jenncarson.com.